"Deep, thoughtful, and practical, this books explores every wave and corner of the cognitive behavioral tradition in search of the best available methods to empower cancer patients. Not content merely to create a jumbled pile of possibilities, Scott Temple lays out a balanced clinical model that makes sense of old and new methods. The years of devotion put into this effort are evident on every page. While a must read if you work with cancer patients, all CBT clinicians will benefit greatly from it, regardless of wave or corner."
Steven C. Hayes, PhD, foundation professor of psychology, University of Nevada

"Dr. Temple has written a moving and meaningful book. His humanity and empathy shine through in his writing. Setting aside the considerable utility of the text in describing work with such patients, the work also masterfully explains the key principles of modern-day CBT and incorporates perspectives from ACT, DBT, and MBCT that amplify and enhance the original model. Vivid case examples and clear summaries make the principles easy to grasp; this is a must read!"
Donna M. Sudak, MD, professor of psychiatry, senior associate training director, and director of psychotherapy training at the Drexel University College of Medicine and past president of the Academy of Cognitive Therapy

"This book provides a unique blend of scholarly and clinical information on all aspects of cognitive behavioral therapy. It is extremely well written and thoroughly edited. I greatly enjoyed reading it, and I strongly recommend this book to all healthcare professionals involved in the care of patients with cancer."
Eduardo Bruera, MD, FT McGraw Chair in the Treatment of Cancer and chair of the Department of Palliative, Rehabilitation and Integrative Medicine at the University of Texas MD Anderson Cancer Center

"In this excellent book, Dr. Temple gives invaluable clinical guidance to those suffering from cancer. His expert advice is rooted in modern CBT and delivered in a compassionate and engaging style. This makes it an important, much needed, and enduring contribution to the literature. The many worksheets, case conceptualizations, and case examples provide patients with concrete tools to relieve some of the suffering and despair. I highly recommend it."

Stefan G. Hofmann, PhD, professor of psychological and brain sciences at Boston University and author of *Emotion in Therapy: From Science to Practice*

"Integrating the best of traditional models of CBT with exciting new developments in the field to develop a coherent treatment approach is no easy project, especially when focusing on the multifaceted issue of cancer. Scott Temple has masterfully accomplished this task, providing a guide that is based in solid theory and research while being clinically useful and highly accessible. This book will be an invaluable resource for any health professional helping people cope with cancer."

James D. Herbert, PhD, dean, executive vice provost, and professor of psychology at the Drexel University Graduate College

"Helping cancer patients face their psychological suffering is a huge challenge. Based on a sound case conceptualization principle, Scott Temple addresses this challenge in the best conceivable manner, bringing to therapists of any persuasion a clear and organized text integrates perspectives from the traditional Beckian CBT and the newer CBT approaches and is richly illustrated with case vignettes. This book offers a compassionate view of those suffering from cancer. I highly recommend it."

Irismar Reis de Oliveira, MD, PhD, professor of psychiatry in the Department of Neuroscience and Mental Health at the Federal University of Bahia, Brazil, and founding fellow of the Academy of Cognitive Therapy

Brief Cognitive Behavior Therapy for Cancer Patients

Brief Cognitive Behavior Therapy for Cancer Patients: Re-Visioning the CBT Paradigm is a practical, clinical guide that allows for the integration of techniques from multiple newer CBT models, organized around a clear conceptual foundation and case conceptualization. The book targets those cognitive, emotional, and behavioral processes that research suggests are instrumental in the maintenance of human psychological suffering. Author Scott Temple also draws on newer models that build on strengths and resilience and brings clinical work to life through vivid case examples, worksheets, and case conceptualization forms. Detailed vignettes show clinicians how to create a case conceptualization as a guide to treatment as well as how to integrate Beckian and newer CBT techniques.

Scott Temple, PhD, is clinical professor and director of psychosocial treatments in the Department of Psychiatry at the University of Iowa. He is on the faculty in the Holden Comprehensive Cancer Center at the University of Iowa and is also a founding fellow and a certified CBT trainer and consultant in the Academy of Cognitive Therapy.

Brief Cognitive Behavior Therapy for Cancer Patients

Re-Visioning the CBT Paradigm

SCOTT TEMPLE

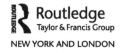

Routledge
Taylor & Francis Group

NEW YORK AND LONDON

First published 2017
by Routledge
711 Third Avenue, New York, NY 10017

and by Routledge
2 Park Square, Milton Park, Abingdon, Oxon, OX14 4RN

Routledge is an imprint of the Taylor & Francis Group, an informa business

Library of Congress Cataloging-in-Publication Data
Names: Temple, Scott, 1948– author.
Title: Brief cognitive behavior therapy for cancer patients : re-visioning the CBT
    paradigm / Scott Temple.
Description: New York, NY : Routledge, 2017. | Includes bibliographical references
    and index.
Identifiers: LCCN 2016015667 | ISBN 9781138942622 (hardback : alk. paper) |
    ISBN 9781138942639 (pbk. : alk. paper) | ISBN 9781315670768 (ebook)
Subjects: | MESH: Cognitive Therapy | Neoplasms—psychology
Classification: LCC RC489.C63 | NLM WM 425.5.C6 | DDC 616.89/1425—dc23
LC record available at https://lccn.loc.gov/2016015667

ISBN: 978-1-138-94262-2 (hbk)
ISBN: 978-1-138-94263-9 (pbk)
ISBN: 978-1-315-67076-8 (ebk)

Typeset in Minion
by Apex CoVantage, LLC

Contents

Acknowledgments

A deep bow to the many generous master clinicians, researchers, and teachers from whom I have learned CBT, ACT, family therapy, brief psychotherapy, and Japanese psychotherapies over the years: Aaron "Tim" Beck, Ivan Boszormenyi-Nagy, Catherine Ducommun-Nagy, James P. Gustafson, Steve Hayes, Marion Lindblad-Goldberg, David K. Reynolds, Steve Simms, and Kelly Wilson. My thanks also to James Bennett-Levy, Trent Codd, Donna Sudak, Kelly Koerner, Brad Beach, Leslie Sokol, and Frank Wills.

My thanks to colleagues at the University of Iowa, in the Department of Psychiatry, and in the Holden Comprehensive Cancer Center. A special thanks to Bev Klug, director of the University of Iowa Mindfulness Programs. Above all, I extend my gratitude to the many patients and families in the Holden Comprehensive Cancer Center at the University of Iowa, who have trusted me to accompany them on their journey in life, and in some cases, their deaths. Names and other relevant identifying material were changed, and in some cases composites are presented in the book, in hopes of preserving the anonymity of patients.

Iowa City is a writer's city, one of the best places in the United States to learn and hone the craft of writing. My thanks to Paul Diehl and Chris Offutt, and to the young writers in the seminars and workshops I was privileged to join in Iowa's fiction and non-fiction programs, many of whom have gone on to publish beautiful stories, novels, and non-fiction works. Finally, I am grateful to my editors at the Routledge/Taylor Frances Group: Anna Moore and Zoey Peresman, whose support, encouragement, and keen editorial eyes have made this a delightful writing experience for me.

To my Soto Zen teacher, Reverend Zuiko Redding, at the Cedar Rapids Zen Center, for her patience, and for teaching me that Samurai leave their swords and their armor at the Zendo door.

Foremost, to Rachel, for 43 years of co-exploring what love, loyalty, forgiveness, and devotion is all about. Thank you, Rachel, for taking care of Lily, our whippet puppy, while I was writing! Now it's my turn.

Introduction

Roughly 1 in 3 Americans will, at some point, develop cancer: whether it is our loved ones, or us, cancer has a high probability of affecting all our lives. Nearly 600,000 Americans will die of cancer each year (American Cancer Society, 2014; Stewart & Wild, 2014). Of those who have cancer, one third or more will experience clinically significant distress (Mitchell et al., 2011, 2012; Levin & Applebaum, 2012). Rates of depression in cancer patients have been estimated to be three times higher than in the general population (Waraich et al., 2004; Li et al., 2012). Clinically significant anxiety may affect as many as 34% of cancer patients (Brintzenhofe-Szoc et al., 2009; Traeger et al., 2012). Those diagnosed with cancer are twice as likely to commit suicide at some point (Misono et al., 2008).

For many of our patients, the shock of a cancer diagnosis is just the beginning of what can be a bewildering and frightening journey, with consequences and demands that require a psychological flexibility that may flag at times, or give out. Relationships, which in some cases may be fragile, are pushed sometimes beyond their limits of sustainability. Changes in physical appearance, from surgery or from the effects of radiation and chemotherapy, lead many to wonder who the person is that they see in the mirror. Sexual functioning may be altered. Fatigue may be omnipresent. Pain may be a constant traveler in the journey, as is the specter of a foreshortened future. Social contacts that were once sustaining may be burdensome now. For patients who are seen with Stage IV disease, metastatic illness, prolongation of life, and preservation of quality of life may be paramount concerns, while hope is maintained that new treatments may come on line in time for them. For those facing, in addition, loss of income, limited life insurance for survivors, no money for transportation and housing, and young children who may be without a parent, the burden of suffering may increase exponentially. One's sense of self may be altered by a diagnosis of cancer. The core beliefs, rules, and assumptions by which one has explicitly or implicitly lived life, and which one assumes govern how life works, may be challenged. The specter of death looms.

And yet, with improved treatments, nearly 65% of cancer patients can expect to live for 5 years and beyond (Stanton et al., 2015). Today, there are nearly 15 million Americans who are in varying phases of survivorship, quadruple that of 30 years ago (American Cancer Society, 2012). They, too, may experience the challenges of re-entry into their daily lives, following treatment. These challenges may include long-term fatigue, pain, role changes, changes in body image, an altered sense of self, impaired sexual functioning, potential cognitive impairments, altered financial status, and changed family relationships. Managing the uncertainty of a future recurrence is sometimes made more challenging as the date of their return clinic visits approach, with intervals extending from perhaps monthly to annually, for the rest of their lives. And finally, the long-term negative effects of treatment itself—surgery, chemotherapy, and radiation therapy—pose additional risks and adaptive challenges. With an eye on managing the psychological needs of the future, Stanton et al. (2015) noted that "a 37% rise in the U.S. population living for 5 or more years with a diagnosis is expected over the next decade" (p. 160).

As I will describe in subsequent chapters, a sense of loss and entrapment, with a breakdown in problem-solving abilities, can contribute to the higher rates of depression and anxiety disorders seen among cancer patients. Those already vulnerable to emotional turbulence, by virtue of prior episodes of depression and adverse childhood experiences, may be especially prone to depression, anxiety, suicidality, and adaptive difficulties in the face of cancer (Williams, M. et al., 2015).

It is a testament to human resilience, however, that most of us find a path through life's greatest challenges. And, in fact, while the rates of depression and anxiety disorders are higher in cancer patients, most people with cancer navigate the challenges of the disease without distress or functional impairments that require the intervention of psychologists and psychiatrists. Those patients with histories of strong adaptive functioning and strong social supports may more easily find that path, though their lives may be forever changed by cancer. And they may need either no services from behavioral health specialists, or need no more than brief, limited encounters. Some will find benefits in the midst of adversity, and the experience of cancer will serve as an opportunity to find renewed meaning and purpose in life (Antoni et al., 2001; Carver & Antoni, 2004). For them, newer CBT innovations address psychological growth and well-being, not just the traditional focus on treating psychological disorders.

Any healer working in a cancer clinic is at times humbled by the strength, the dignity, and the resourcefulness of people dealing with life adversity, and on any given day, one might learn as much or more from one's patients as one does from those who serve them. Just as our patients require great resourcefulness to deal with the challenges of cancer, so, too, do treaters need resourcefulness. In addition, we need a strong grounding in the most effective and promising treatments, with the ability to be flexible in our delivery and our techniques, in order to target the most relevant clinical processes in the most humane and heartfelt manner possible. At the same time, our patients require us to grow as healers and as human beings, in a way that allows us to remain open to their pain and ours, genuine in our compassion, while relentlessly inventive in helping them find a way to meet each challenge they face. As one patient put it as we summarized our work, at the conclusion of months of psychotherapy for her Stage IV bladder cancer, now in apparent remission: "This has been like a pillar for me, a place where I can talk, solve problems, and get comfort."

Here is a look at an afternoon in the cancer clinic:

Outpatient Cancer Clinic
University Hospital
Tuesday, May 5th

1:00 p.m.: Claire Reynolds is a 25-year-old single woman who is recovering from chemotherapy and surgery for Stage III breast cancer. After two good reports, each at 3-month intervals, she is now only scheduled for follow-up at 6 months. And while the reduced monitoring schedule signals her good recovery prospects, she is afraid to spend so much time away from the medical team that saved her life. Faced with good prospects for survival, she is nonetheless distraught and tearful in her first meeting with a psychologist. She fears that any pain might be due to a return of cancer. In line with this, she is beginning to direct her attention and awareness obsessively to her body, to scan herself for signs that something is wrong. In addition, she is now experiencing preoccupations and rituals that make her fear she is losing her mind:

> I know I don't have to worry about germs now that my chemo is done. But I can't stop worrying about getting sick. I am washing my hands after I touch any food, at home, in grocery stores. My hands are getting red, and it's embarrassing.

She stretches out her arms to display the mottled red skin that runs from her fingers to an abrupt line just above the wrists. She has no prior history of obsessive-compulsive disorder: "If I eat at someone's house, I worry about whether the food got contaminated. So I stay home, even though I want to be with people." Her distress increases as she speaks. "I'm afraid I'm losing my mind."

2:00 p.m.: Andrea Woodson is a 50-year-old career woman with no prior history of psychological difficulties or treatment. She is married, without children. A nagging pain in the abdomen developed several months ago and persisted, despite her belief that it would go away of its own accord. When the pain becomes sharp and persistent, she goes to her primary care doctor, who becomes suspicious and sends her to the university cancer center. There, she learns that she has Stage IV pancreatic cancer and that survival prospects are grim. She appears for a first session with her husband, and announces: "I don't need services for myself." Yet the psychologist is concerned that she might benefit, after hearing Andrea state, "This shouldn't be happening to me. I run. I diet. I've looked after my health since I was young. This is not supposed to be happening!"

A moment later, Andrea's affect shifts. "There's something else that's more important right now," she says, now looking at her husband, whose hand she takes. "I am afraid that John will want to kill himself if I die. He said as much." Then, looking back at the psychologist, she states in earnest, "I want you to help keep him alive if and when I don't make it through this."

Her husband looks grimly toward the psychologist but says nothing.

3:00 p.m.: Liz Romano is 26. She is nearly one year out from surgery and radiation therapy for a rare cancerous tumor of the skull. One day, more than a year earlier, her left eye suddenly turned outward. Two harrowing surgeries later, she faced radiation. The good news? She has excellent survival chances, has finished her treatments, and returned to the small town where she lives with her husband and young son. However, resuming her active life as a mother, wife, worker, and amateur athlete has been accompanied by puzzling and disturbing experiences. Each time she has a headache, she is overwhelmed by fear of cancer recurrence. She is now focusing on her body, checking for any signs that something is wrong. This is intruding on her ability to live her life fully. More disturbing, she spontaneously and unpredictably experiences the physical sensations that followed her awakening from anesthetic and her first brain surgery. She feels and imagines the searing pain, radiating from her head, down her spine. She imagines the feelings and the images of vomiting blood. This replay is increasing in frequency, and she is at a loss to understand what is happening. She has never told anyone else about this: "I keep doing everything I need to do in my life, but it is getting harder. Can you help me with this?"

4:00 p.m.: Elvira Mortensen is a 58-year-old woman, married with two adult children and five grandchildren, all living in other parts of the country. She has Stage IV colon cancer, and she realizes that she will eventually die from the disease. She appears in the first session to accept her illness. However, she is concerned about quality of life and this links with her long-standing marital disillusionment. She states that her husband refuses to accept that she has a terminal illness and strongly opposes accommodations to her illness. These include stopping work and the attendant decline in family finances this represents. In addition, she states that he will not help with chores in the house, though she is increasingly disabled by fatigue and pain. She would like to travel while she is still able to visit her children and grandchildren. But, she says, her husband refuses to spend the money, now that she is no longer working: "I don't know what to do," she says, and she begins to cry. "I know I'm going to die from this. But this isn't the way I want to spend however long I have left."

We will return to these cases in subsequent chapters, to show how those cases were conceptualized and what interventions were brought to bear on the task of helping each person. This book will draw on the findings from more recent scientific and clinical advances in the field, to expand the framework for using CBT with cancer patients. While reasonably effective treatments exist, the field has changed, and new findings may lead to improved outcomes for patients.

In his Pulitzer Prize–winning history of cancer, *The Emperor of All Maladies*, Siddhartha Mukherjee (2010) concluded with the case of a dying psychologist. Germaine Berne has a rare gastric cancer. After 5 years of surgeries, chemotherapy, remissions, triumph, and relapse, she faces her death. Mukherjee describes Dr. Berne's elegance, her fierce will to live, her relentless search for a cure or the prolongation of her life, the triumph of her remission, the terror of her disease's return, the compensations made to remain dignified as her body has been increasingly wrecked by disease, and finally the acceptance of her inevitable and impending death.

Years later, reflecting on his last conversation with her before her death, he wrote, "Germaine seemed, that evening, to have captured something essential about our struggle against cancer: that, to keep pace with this malady, you needed to keep inventing and reinventing, learning and unlearning strategies" (Mukherjee, 2010, p. 470). At the conclusion of the PBS series based on his book, *The Emperor of All Maladies*, Siddhartha Mukherjee stated simply, "The cancer cell is evolving. And so are we."

This book is an attempt to take a fresh step in the evolution of our treatments for people with cancer, by incorporating newer developments within CBT, without sacrificing what we know is already helpful. We know that both individual and group administered Cognitive Behavior Therapy has demonstrated efficacy in treating depression and anxiety in cancer patients, though the efficacy is less than perfect (Li et al., 2012).

Why might there be a need for a more integrative effort such as this? The past 20 years have seen an explosion of new theoretical, scientific, and technical advances within the field of Cognitive Behavior Therapy. The introduction of mindfulness and acceptance-based therapies has had an impact on the field (Hayes, 2004; Herbert & Foreman, 2011), and newer ways of understanding the nature and function of cognition have transformed the clinical landscape as well (Hayes et al., 2012; Segal et al., 2013).

The integration of the traditional and the new within Cognitive Behavior Therapy offers the possibility of more carefully honed formulations and a greater breadth of techniques and interventions. This book offers a systematic integration of the old and the new in the field of Cognitive Behavior Therapy, organized around eight key principles for a Modern Cognitive Behavior Therapy. The intent is to allow clinicians to conceptualize cases and to draw on the newest developments in the science and theories of CBT, to relieve suffering and enhance well-being in those we serve. The primary focus will be on the delivery of individual therapy, with as-needed inclusion of partners, family members, and members of the care team. Research on transdiagnostic factors in psychological disorders will be drawn on in a way that helps apply the model to patients who are distressed, yet who are considered sub-syndromal in their depression and anxiety problems.

The focus will be on establishing a robust therapeutic relationship while delivering interventions that offer the most hope of reducing the high levels of distress and suffering encountered by clinicians working with cancer patients.

Cognitive Behavior Therapy (CBT) is more aptly described not as a single therapy but as a family of therapies. Sharing a common commitment to science, the field was rooted initially in behaviorism. Yet by the late 1960s, it was clear behaviorism had not adequately met the challenge of explaining human language and cognition, despite an early attempt by B. F. Skinner to do just that (Skinner, 1957). It would initially fall to Albert Ellis and Aaron Beck to develop clinical models that incorporated behaviorism into a cognitive framework. By the late 1970s, the so-called Cognitive Revolution was in full swing. And with it, CBT would become, by the turn of the century, among the most widely disseminated and empirically validated forms of psychotherapy (Hofmann, 2012).

By no means content to rest on its laurels, the field of CBT sought to understand not only what works in psychotherapy but also why it works. One of the central features of the community of cognitive behavioral therapies is the commitment to understand the basic mechanisms of human suffering and to evolve treatment models that work, based on verifiable theories and principles. We will briefly explore in a subsequent chapter the challenges posed by newer clinical models to Beck's Cognitive Therapy. While we know that Beck's model provides benefit for people suffering from many psychological disorders, the science of CBT has raised intriguing questions about not only why but also how the model might work. Some of the questions, and the findings, have challenged Cognitive Therapy's foundations (Hayes et al., 2012). And this, in turn, has led to exciting newer advances, each potentially extending the range and effectiveness of our treatment efforts.

Among these newer empirically supported therapies are those with roots in ancient and modern contemplative traditions, newer accounts of human information processing, memory, language, and cognition. Others have introduced mindfulness and acceptance, blended with a return to the behavioral core of CBT. Among the more widely known and evidence-based of these therapies are Acceptance and Commitment Therapy (ACT; Hayes, Villatte et al., 2011), Dialectical Behavior Therapy (DBT; Linehan, 1993b; 2015), Metacognitive Therapy (MCT; Wells, 2000; 2009), and Mindfulness-Based Cognitive Therapy (MBCT; Segal et al., 2013; Williams, M. et al., 2015). Each of these models has pioneered new ground in our understanding of human suffering. And each has offered new theoretical and technical innovations to help alleviate that suffering. This includes advances in treating depression, suicide risk, and anxiety disorders. In addition, many of these newer therapies depart from a medical model of human suffering to address issues of meaning and purpose in life. This is perhaps best exemplified by Marsha Linehan's focus on building "a life worth living," using DBT. ACT is built on a core of behaviorism, a new behavioral account of human language, and a goal of helping people achieve the freedom to live in accord with their deepest values in life. MBCT shares with DBT a focus on mindfulness training and practice as a core means of helping people achieve freedom from the tyranny of mental traps and destructive action urges.

In sum, these newer models build on CBT in a way that may help us more effectively meet the many and varied psychological needs of people with cancer. If, as Siddhartha Mukherjee (2010) said, we need "to keep inventing and reinventing, learning and unlearning strategies" (p. 470), these newer models offer us that promise.

Reinventing CBT does not mean discarding what we know works. It means refining and expanding our clinical interventions on the basis of newer scientific findings and evolving treatment models. Problem-Solving Therapy (Nezu et al., 1999; 2007; 2012) and Cognitive Therapy (Moorey & Greer, 2012; Levin et al., 2013; Levin, White, Bialer et al., 2013) already have established an evidence base for use with cancer patients. Newer models have in most cases not been tested adequately, though a form of MBCT has shown initial promise in working with cancer patients (Carlson & Speca, 2010; Bartley, 2012; Rouleau et al., 2015).

This book will provide a theoretically coherent model of CBT that allows flexible integration of techniques from multiple, empirically supported CBT models. I am not unmindful of the challenges of attempting an integration of this sort. Wells and Fisher (2016a), developers of Metacognitive Therapy, warned that blending techniques and principles of various CBT models can lead to confusion, diminished efficacy, and a departure from the scientific basis of each model. A focus on cognitive content, for example, can be theoretically incompatible with a focus on cognitive processes, as noted by adherents of MBCT, MCT, and ACT. And blending Beckian and so-called "Third Wave" approaches can engender confusion in patients and therapists. But I do not believe such problems are inevitable, and I would suggest that the principles outlined in this book allow for effective technical integration. If the technical focus is integrative here, the case conceptualization is rooted in new developments in Beck's model of Cognitive Therapy (Persons, 1989; 2008; J. Beck, 1995; 2011a; Brewin, 2006; Kuyken et al., 2009; Westbrook et al., 2012; Wills & Sanders, 2013; Bennett-Levy et al., 2015; Wills, 2015). The aim will be to maintain the commitment that all CBT therapies have for clinical and scientific rigor while presenting a model that is immediately useful for clinicians, trainees, and researchers in the field. The key features of this model include the following organizing principles:

1.   Normalizing human suffering;
2.   Balancing acceptance, mindfulness, and change processes;
3.   A focus on transdiagnostic processes in psychological disorders;
4.   Balancing cognitive and experiential interventions in CBT;
5.   An increased focus on self-processes in therapy;
6.   A more contextual model of human functioning;
7.   A focus on strengths, resilience, and well-being;
8.   The disciplined use of the therapist's self in fostering the treatment relationship.

Chapter Outlines and Chapter Organization

Part I of this book provides a brief overview of theory and research. Chapter 1 presents the psychological and physical challenges that cancer patients face, from the time of diagnosis and early treatment through survivorship. Chapter 2 describes the clinical principles in the model to be employed with cases throughout the book. The chapter will emphasize the importance of a principle-driven approach to treatment, rather than one that is more rigidly manualized, allowing the inter-related principles to be flexibly applied in the service of meeting the patient where they are. Research will be briefly summarized, leading to the model of human suffering and therapeutic techniques described in subsequent chapters. Chapter 3 details the opening moves in establishing an effective treatment relationship as well as strategies for boosting the relationship. A collaborative and emotionally evocative treatment will be described, with an eye toward developing and honing one's relationship-building strategies, utilizing Beck's Guided Discovery and Socratic Questioning (GD/SQ) and Linehan's DBT's validation strategies.

Chapter 4 provides a description of how to create case formulations, which guide treatment. The establishment of treatment targets will be described, on the basis of identifying the relevant psychological and interpersonal processes that have become problematic. In particular, an emphasis will be given to rapid formulations, necessitated by what are often brief therapy encounters in cancer clinics. The second part of the chapter addresses the issue of how to structure of an effective CBT session.

Part Two of the book details the clinical applications of the CBT model described in Part One. The emphasis will be on relatively brief therapy, tailored to the needs of patients presenting in clinical cancer centers. Although many such patients present in acute distress, their phase of cancer can range from newly diagnosed to treatment, relapse, or varying stages of survivorship. Applications of the model for patients at all phases, and experiencing depression, anxiety, and life problems, will be demonstrated.

Chapter 5 addresses the treatment of depression in cancer patients and utilizes new advances in our understanding of depression. Depression occurring in the context of multiple prior depressive episodes as well as adverse childhood experiences will be addressed. Core processes of rumination, withdrawal, and restricted problem-solving skills will be a focus of the chapter. Chapter 6 focuses on the assessment and treatment of depression in cancer patients, including sub-syndromal presentations. Chapter 7 focuses primarily on treating anxiety problems in cancer patients, including management of acute fear states, chronic worry states, avoidance, and helplessness. The chapter focuses on anxiety problems that impede engagement in cancer therapy as well as anxiety problems occurring in the various survivorship phases.

Chapter 8 describes a very brief treatment focus, intended to put a floor under the distressed cancer patient. The emphasis will be on clinical work with patients newly diagnosed, experiencing a psychological crisis in the context of treatment, or when dealing with recurrence or metastatic illness.

Chapter 9 addresses therapist self-care and self-practice. We will explore the use of the principles of treatment for the care of the therapist as well as the care team. Opportunities to identify beliefs that can undermine effective management of self in relation to ill patients will be provided. Emotion management strategies and the cultivation of perspective-taking skills and compassion practices will be described. The clinician will have an opportunity to employ the principles in the book to develop a self-care plan and set of practices that can minimize exposure to burnout. In addition, the role of the oncology team as a consultation team to one another will be described.

Since the intended audience will be experienced clinicians, teachers, supervisors, and trainees from a variety of disciplines, clinical chapters will contain ample opportunities to learn therapy in action. Case descriptions will be provided, with case vignettes and therapy transcripts included. Readers will have the chance to see how the case conceptualization shifts as new information arises in session, how interventions are formed, and how to respond when interventions succeed and when they fail. Case examples from various phases of cancer treatment and recovery will be used to illustrate principles. All cases are disguised to protect confidentiality, though they represent actual clinical situations that clinicians may encounter in their practices. Most chapters will contain an end-of-chapter summary and/or key points.

Part I
Theory and Research

One
The Psychosocial and Physical Challenges of Cancer

The literature on the psychological, interpersonal, and physical challenges posed by cancer is voluminous and has grown exponentially since the early 1970s, when Jimmie Holland, MD, pioneered the field of psycho-oncology at Memorial Sloan Kettering Cancer Center (Holland, 2002). At the same time, Moorey and Greer (2012) began the development of Cognitive Behavior Therapy for cancer, on the basis of early literature regarding the psychosocial impact of cancer. For our purposes, it may be useful to categorize the literature, and our treatment formulations, on the basis of the following:

1. The most commonly occurring psychological and adaptive difficulties associated with cancer,
2. The phase of treatment and survivorship of the cancer patient,
3. Adapting for site and stage of cancer as well as effects of both the cancer and treatment,
4. Use of a CBT case conceptualization to tailor the formulation to the specific idiographic needs of each patient.

Moorey and Greer (2012) outlined the psychological and interpersonal challenges that a diagnosis of cancer creates. These responses may include an initial sense of shock and disbelief, as one begins to process the meaning of cancer as a potential existential threat. Cancer, in the CBT model employed by Moorey and Greer, threatens the core beliefs, rules, and assumptions that have explicitly and implicitly guided the person in his or her daily life. A diagnosis of cancer can threaten the entire system of meaning by which one's life is organized. Drawing on the work of Lazarus and Folkmann (1984), they described responses to stress as affected by the person's appraisals of the situation. Moorey and Greer (2012) focused on how the person's appraisals of the threat posed by cancer can be organized into what they describe as five adjustment styles:

1. Fighting spirit
2. Avoidance or denial
3. Fatalism
4. Helplessness and hopelessness
5. Anxious preoccupation.

The person who sees illness as a challenge to be managed exemplifies a *fighting spirit*. Such people seek information, are actively engaged in their treatment and recovery processes, and refrain from dwelling via rumination and unproductive worry. As one patient described, "We are a family that believes in playing the cards we're dealt. And we play them as well as possible."

Avoidance or denial may be a way of keeping intense fear states at bay, but it comes at a price. By not facing the emotional impact of the disease, the person may cut himself or herself off from valuable sources of information from within. In addition, avoidance and denial can prevent the patient from not only facing "the cards they are dealt" but also engaging in effective problem-solving behaviors and from being meaningful collaborators in their own care. *Fatalism* is essentially a passive stance toward illness and illness management. It may superficially resemble acceptance, but true acceptance is a form of engagement, from which spring forth adaptive responses to life's challenges. Fatalism, on the other hand, tends not to lead to active adaptive responses, where such responses are indicated and warranted. In *helplessness and hopelessness*, the patient is overwhelmed and simply gives up. This is a classically depressive response. *Anxious preoccupation* is characterized by prolonged worry states and maladaptive reassurance seeking. We will see in Chapter 7 on treatment of cancer-related anxiety that an understanding of both cognitive biases and maladaptive cognitive processes and coping strategies inform treatment efforts.

In addition to Moorey and Greer's Beckian CBT model, Problem-Solving Therapy (PST) is an empirically supported treatment. PST adds to the understanding of how people with cancer cope with a diagnosis and treatment of cancer, by referring to the person's problem orientation (Nezu et al., 1999; Nezu et al., 2007). The Nezus have categorized the person's problem orientation in terms of the following:

1. *Positive problem orientation*, in which problems are seen as a normal, expectable part of life. Problems are viewed as challenges to be solved or mastered, and the person views himself or herself as capable of dealing with life's problems. The person recognizes that persistence and effort are required to solve problems, and that engagement, rather than avoidance, is required.

2. *Negative problem orientation* occurs when problems are viewed as large, unsolvable threats, with the person lacking the resources to manage the threat effectively. The person may become prone to emotion dysregulation in the face of problems, leading to the use of ineffective problem-solving styles, as follows.

In addition, they have described three problem-solving styles, one of which is effective:

1. *Rational problem-solving style,* which is a systematic and deliberate strategy of engagement;
2. *Impulsivity/carelessness style,* which involves seeing few solutions to a problem and impulsively selecting one without thinking through the consequences;
3. *Avoidance style,* characterized by passivity, denial, avoidance, and reliance on others to solve the problem.

While there are data supporting the efficacy of these two approaches, the relationship between problem orientations/adjustment styles and cancer outcome is equivocal. Hopelessness and helplessness are associated with poorer disease outcome, while the more active, engaged styles and orientations do not necessarily ensure improved cancer outcome (Garssen, 2004). Promoting a more engaged style of coping may nonetheless improve quality of life and reduce the burden of psychological distress.

The data regarding depression and anxiety disorders in newly diagnosed and treated cancer patients have revealed considerable variability in prevalence estimates. Levin and Kissane (2006) reported that major depression may occur in 10% to 25% of cancer patients. Li et al. (2012) reported major depression in approximately 16% of cancer patients. However, distress from depression symptoms can be significant, even if the patient does not meet the more restrictive criteria for major depressive disorder (MDD). And if we use depressive symptoms rather than MDD as our criteria, up to 58% of cancer patients may report depressive symptoms (Massie, 2004). Li et al. (2012) reported minor depression and dysthymia in 22% of cancer patients. Since fatigue and appetite problems can result from cancer and cancer treatment and not just from depression, it is worth teasing out these processes. When doing so, and substituting cognitive symptoms for fatigue and appetite difficulties, depressive rates are unchanged (Trask, 2004; Levin & Kissane, 2006). It is likely that when employing *Diagnostic and Statistical Manual of Mental Disorders (DSM)* criteria, the prevalence of depression in cancer patients may be twice that of the general U.S. population (Jacobsen & Andrykowski, 2015). And, suicide is twice as likely to occur in cancer patients than in those without cancer (Misono et al., 2008). It is clinically important to recognize that cancer-related depression "is associated with fewer core depressive thoughts, such as a sense of guilt and failure, dissatisfaction and self-dislike, than primary depression" (Li et al., 2012, p. 1188). In addition, the prevalence of depression in cancer patients is equally distributed between men and women, unlike the roughly 2:1 male:female prevalence of depression in the general population, possibly due to the more even split of the disease's occurrence (Li et al., 2012).

Similar variability exists in prevalence of anxiety problems in cancer patients, with rates ranging from 0.9% to 49% (van't Spijer et al., 1997). Levin and Kissane (2006) described estimates ranging from 15% to 28%, using the Hospital Anxiety and Depression Scales. Mitchell et al. (2011) placed the prevalence of anxiety disorders in cancer patients at 10.3%. A study of adult outpatients in a large cancer center has shown that 34% of patients reported significant problems with anxiety (Brintzenhofe-Szoc et al., 2009). Sub-syndromal anxiety can be quite distressing and may be related to situational and/or existential concerns, such as panic occurring in cancer patients who have young, dependent children (Traeger et al., 2012). Anxiety problems can be transient or episodic, such as anxiety associated with upcoming procedures or outpatient return visits for monitoring by the oncology team. Vulnerability to anxiety disorders is increased by having a history of anxiety disorders prior to the onset of cancer, though medical phobias, features of post-traumatic stress disorder, panic, and worry are quite possible in the absence of a prior history of anxiety disorders.

Clinically significant anxiety and depressive problems are the psychological problems most likely to occur in newly diagnosed and treated patients as well as those with newly diagnosed recurrences (Jacobsen & Andrykowski, 2015). Factors affecting the presence of depression include hopelessness, lack of social support, a prior history of depression, and adverse childhood experiences. It is also possible that the biology of cancer, in some cases, such as pancreatic cancer, may also confer risk for depression. Similarly, some chemotherapy treatments, too, may induce depression (Jacobsen & Andrykowski, 2015). Steroids can be implicated in depression in cancer patients, as can some immunotherapies (Musselman et al., 2001). Stage of cancer is less predictive of depression, anxiety, or distress than one might expect (Levin & Kissane, 2006).

Difficulties with estimating prevalence rates of depressive and anxiety disorders reflect measurement issues as well as differentiating between distress occurring in syndromal versus sub-syndromal depression and anxiety. A more common approach to screening has involved assessing global distress, rather than beginning by seeking a *DSM* diagnosis. When using simple visual analog scales or thermometers, patients can be simply and quickly screened in a way that correlates well with more formal psychiatric assessments, such as the Hospital Anxiety and Depression Scale (HADS), and identifies up to 19% of patients as a concern (Jacobsen et al., 2005; Levin & Kissane, 2006). Distress alone, however, is an imperfect indicator of a need for referral to a behavioral health clinician. Many distressed patients experience a reduction in their distress over the course of cancer treatment, suggesting that distress at the time of an initial diagnosis is not necessarily a predictor of a need for psychological services (Salmon et al., 2015). In addition, patients newly diagnosed with cancer are customarily distressed, yet may be highly resistant to focusing on their emotional reactions (Baker et al., 2013).

In addition to the psychological effects of being diagnosed and treated for cancer, there are physical effects of cancer and cancer treatment, which intertwine with and influence adaptive behavior and coping. The most common physical effects are fatigue and pain. Between 60% and 90% of patients in treatment for cancer may report clinically significant fatigue (Flechtner & Bottomley, 2003), with fatigue continuing to be a potential problem for years after the completion of treatment. CBT has demonstrated efficacy in managing the effects of fatigue and pain in cancer patients (Jacobsen & Andrykowski, 2015). Significant pain, for example, affects perhaps 25% to 33% of patients (Jacobsen & Andrykowski, 2015). The causes and maintaining factors in cancer pain are complex and include the disease site and severity; the use of surgical, radiation, or chemotherapies, and psychological factors that contribute to pain. The latter include a tendency toward a catastrophizing cognitive response, hopelessness, isolation, and withdrawal, in addition to anxious arousal and worry. The response of caregivers to pain may also serve as a maintaining factor for pain.

The number of patients surviving 5 years or more after a cancer diagnosis has grown steadily over the past 35 years and will continue to do so. Estimates have suggested "a 37% rise in the U.S. population living for 5 or more years with a cancer diagnosis is expected over the next decade" (Stanton et al., 2015, p. 160). Thus, by 2022, 67% of the estimated 18 million people diagnosed with cancer will survive beyond 5 years (deMoor et al., 2013). The service needs for this large number of people will be extraordinary. In addition, we will need to evolve our service models in order to address the challenges that cancer patients and their families will face throughout the long and changing course of survivorship. Part of that challenge will involve helping people adjust to the possible long-term consequences of cancer and cancer treatment: fatigue, pain, body image changes, changes in sexual functioning, family impact, work and income effects, and changes in one's sense of meaning and purpose in life.

Patients who are in the survivorship phase, which begins at treatment completion, have their own commonly occurring challenges, which may vary over the course of survivorship. (Stanton et al., 2015) conceptualized survivorship as containing three broad phases or stages:

1. The re-entry phase, extending from the end of treatment to roughly two years after diagnosis;
2. Early survivorship, from 2 to 5 years post diagnosis;
3. Long-term survivorship, from 5 years post diagnosis and beyond.

The authors were careful to indicate that theirs is a rough heuristic and that the course of survivorship is not yet fully understood. But the heuristic (see Figure 1.1) is nonetheless useful in conceptualizing problems and in organizing our treatment efforts with patients who are post treatment.

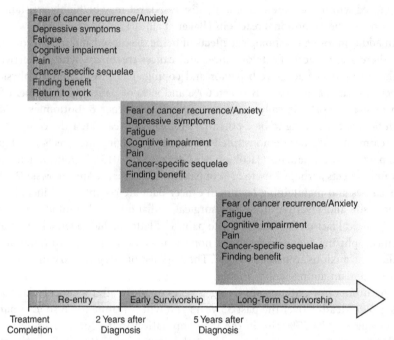

FIGURE 1.1 Hypothesized Periods of Cancer Survivorship and Associated Sequelae: An Evolving Heuristic Model

Source: Stanton et al. (2015). Life after diagnosis and treatment of cancer in adulthood: contributions from psychosocial oncology research. *American Psychologist*, 70 (2), p. 161.

Figure 1.1 organizes phases of survivorship and points the clinician to commonly occurring challenges and protective factors in these phases. This, in turn, helps us organize our assessment and clinical inquiry and target relevant problems. The re-entry phase can be viewed as a time when treatment ends, and the patient no longer requires such frequent contact with the cancer treatment team. Re-entry into daily life can include a return to work, with whatever limitations are imposed by the illness and by the effects of treatment. The patient faces the need to adjust expectations and performance accordingly. In addition, the patient's support network may have mobilized for the treatment phase and may be less prepared for the sometimes slow pace of recovery. This may be especially true when cancer pain and fatigue linger. Depressive irritability, withdrawal, and anxiety all can affect not only the patient but also his or her social network, setting up vicious cycles of interactions that may deepen depression and anxiety. Finally, the end of treatment can be accompanied by an increase of fear and worry, as the patient loses frequent contact with the medical team. During re-entry, the patient can become more focused on physical sensations and symptoms, which can in turn be interpreted in a catastrophic light, leading to health anxiety when the medical team is not available for frequent reassurance and support (Stanton et al., 2015).

In essence, the medical team can become a safety behavior (Salkovskis, 1996a), and the patient's dependence on the team for reassurance can be counterproductive. Psychoeducation, with opportunities to adjust expectations for recovery, can be a vital intervention when patients and families may otherwise hold unrealistic expectations for life after treatment.

In the early survivorship phase, after re-entry, patients may experience upsurges in anxiety as they return for monitoring, in anticipation of whether they will learn of a recurrence of illness. This customarily occurs during the early survivorship phase, roughly up to about 5 years post diagnosis. During this phase, depression, fatigue, anxiety problems, and pain may continue as well as the specific sequelae of the patient's unique cancer and treatment profile, including possible cognitive impairments. Long-term survivorship remains prone to worry about recurrence, although depression prospects diminish. However, the long-term effects of cancer and cancer treatment may be pronounced, and they are becoming more prominent as more patients enter long-term survivorship.

Among the possible sequelae of cancer, across all phases of survivorship, are the following:

1. Fear of recurrence/anxiety
2. Fatigue
3. Cognitive impairment
4. Cancer-specific sequelae (depending upon primary site, staging, treatment)
5. Finding benefit.

Stanton et al. (2015) hypothesized depression to be more likely during the first 5 years of survivorship. If the patient experiences a recurrence during survivorship, they become vulnerable to depression and anxiety. In fact, those with second cancers may be even more likely to experience clinically significant depression and anxiety problems than they did during the initial episode of cancer (Jacobsen & Andrykowski, 2015).

It is important to note that in the natural course of adapting to cancer or other serious illnesses, people discover that positive changes have occurred, and that disease has brought with it unanticipated benefits. This process is sometimes described as "benefit finding" (Jacobsen & Andrykowski, 2015). Cancer is also seen as creating a potential "teachable moment," which Stanton et al. (2015) described as "a life transition or event, which can motivate individuals to adopt risk-reducing or health-enhancing behaviors" (p. 165). Another term sometimes used is "post-traumatic growth" (Tedeschi & Calhoun, 1996, p. 455). These processes often occur spontaneously, with between 50% and 80% of post-treatment cancer survivors experiencing such benefits (Stanton et al., 2006; Jacobsen & Andrykowski, 2015). Stanton et al. (2015) stated that "key domains of self-reported benefit include strengthened interpersonal relationships, commitment to life priorities, life appreciation, personal regard, spirituality, and attention to health behaviors."

In addition, they noted that "longitudinal research suggest that finding benefit increases from the diagnostic and treatment phase through the reentry and early survivorship phase" (p. 165).

It is an irony of the human experience that such growth may require, or at least be propelled by, the very pain that we most seek to avoid in life. This irony, and the attendant power of growth in the midst of pain, has been recognized for millennia, and has been immortalized in the writings of our greatest dramatists, poets, and spiritual teachers. The Greek tragedian and playwright Aeschylus likely experienced his own post-traumatic growth after fighting as an Athenian soldier in the Battle of Marathon, 2,500 years ago. Aeschylus's most poignant words deeply affected and sustained Robert F. Kennedy in the months and years following the assassination of his older brother. Those words spontaneously came to his mind as Kennedy prepared the speech he would give to a primarily African American audience in Indianapolis, on the night of Martin Luther King, Jr.'s death. Kennedy said,

> My favorite poet was Aeschylus. He once wrote, 'And even in our sleep, pain which cannot forget falls drop by drop upon the heart, until in our own despair, against our will, comes wisdom through the awful grace of God.'

Pain is the one teacher that none of us wants; it can also be the one teacher from which we can learn our most important lessons about living. This spontaneous human capacity to find benefits and growth opportunities in the midst of pain is a fortuitous ally in our treatment efforts. We want to listen and watch for this, so that we can ride with the patient into these teachable moments for finding benefits and growth. One CBT model that is poised to contribute to this effort is Acceptance and Commitment Therapy (ACT), which places values front and center in its model. One clinical trial of ACT for colorectal survivors has suggested that ACT can contribute to improved psychosocial outcomes in just the processes that Stanton et al. (2006) described as subject to spontaneous post-cancer growth: spiritual growth, renewed commitment to life priorities, life appreciation, strengthened relationships, personal regard, and health behaviors. These changes in spiritual growth and other values increased over the course of 1-year follow-up and appear to be partially mediated by acceptance and mindfulness processes (Hawkes et al., 2013; Hawkes et al., 2014).

ACT has vividly described the ways in which pain and values are deeply intertwined with one another. An ACT dictum reads that "in your pain lie your values," and this becomes immediately evident when working with people who have cancer. To wit:

Over the course of a month, three different men, each with a different form of cancer, each from different walks of life, in different phases of life, at different points in their treatments, and with different prospects for recovery, each said the same thing to me: "I wish I'd been a better husband. I wish I'd been there for her." In each case, their predicaments brought them face-to-face with how deeply they cherished their wives and how deeply each believed they had wounded or been distant from their wives during their marriages. Whether through previous affairs, or too much time spent at work, having been emotionally remote, too focused on hobbies when away from work, or inattentive to the financial protection they hoped to provide, these men all said the same thing. In sorting through their beliefs and the histories of their marriages, we reached the same conclusion in each case: no matter how much time remained, the present moment provided an opportunity to be the husband they would wish to be, now.

We can now conceptualize cancer and its treatment, for our purposes, using the following timeline and processes. These phases and challenges begin with diagnosis and continue throughout either the long-term process of survivorship or end-of-life and palliative care treatment:

1. Initial diagnosis and early treatment phase;
2. Treatment phase: curative, uncertain, non-curative;
3. Survivorship and monitoring: re-entry, early survivorship, long-term survivorship;
4. Palliative care and end-of-life concerns.

Figure 1.2 provides a flow chart for treatment, and possible outcomes, with commonly occurring problematic and non-problematic processes included.

Treatment efforts need to be organized around a framework that derives from an understanding of the challenges and potential difficulties associated with every phase of cancer care, from the initial diagnosis to long-term survivorship, to possible end-of-life care. This heuristic can assist the psycho-oncology team in organizing care, on the basis of the awareness of where a patient fits into this schema. The heuristic allows for a highly flexible and idiographic case formulation to be derived, unique to each patient and their interpersonal network. The latter will be developed in Chapter 4 on case formulations.

Let's now return to cases from our introduction, and two others, to place them along the continuum shown in Figure 1.2.

Our 1:00 p.m. clinic patient, 25-year-old Claire Reynolds, can be described as in *the re-entry phase* of recovery. Given her Stage III breast cancer, we cannot yet know what her long-term survival prospects are. With the reduction in daily contact with the treatment team, now to include monitoring at 6-month intervals, she is fearful. She is scrutinizing her body for signals that her cancer may have returned, and since she does not see her oncologist now for many months, her fears amplify as she worries and directs attentional resources to physical cues that signal something is terribly wrong. Worse still, she is now obsessing about germ exposure, a likely holdover of her immunosuppressed state during chemotherapy. And again, she has no one on the medical team with whom to talk about her fears. Finally, work, finances, and social support are problematic now, complicating her re-entry.

Our 2:00 p.m. patient, 50-year-old Andrea Woodson, is facing *end-of-life issues*, with her Stage IV pancreatic cancer as well as dealing with the new diagnosis of

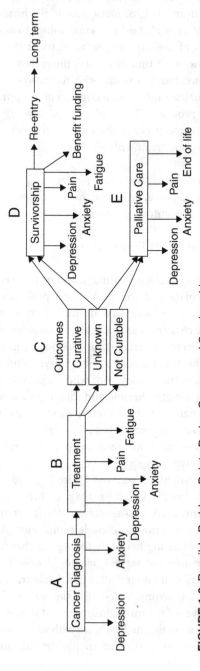

FIGURE 1.2 Possible Problem Points During Cancer and Survivorship

cancer. Although one can safely surmise that she has many concerns about how her remaining time will pass, including pain management, how her body might shut down, how much time she has left, and many other potential concerns, today her primary concern is for her husband. She fears for him, because she knows that her untimely death will be potentially devastating for him, perhaps leading to a suicidal crisis, which she asks the psychologist to help avert. Andrea has a very strong history of adaptive functioning and problem-solving strengths. She is methodical and effective in her thinking and her stance toward life challenges. At the same time, the current situation she faces is exceptionally painful, and while she indicates that she can find a path through facing the terminal illness she now has, she needs help in solving the one challenge for which she will not be alive to manage: her husband's response to her death.

Our 3:00 p.m. patient, Liz Romano, 26, is now in *the early survivorship phase*, 2 years out from diagnosis and beginning treatment. The treatment was highly invasive and frightening for her, and she has features of post-traumatic stress disorder, which have not resolved with time. She has made a successful return to work. She is an active wife and mother. And she has resumed her play in summer women's softball leagues. She lives in a small town, at a considerable distance from the university cancer center, and is infrequently monitored. While the medical news is very good, she is isolated from the sources of information and help that the oncology team might otherwise provide, and her family is frightened by the re-living experiences and nightmares she endures. Liz has a strong history of adaptive functioning and, in many ways, has triumphed in her management of deeply traumatic surgery and chemotherapy. The upsurge of troubling post-traumatic stress-related problems is bewildering to her. She has no language for understanding what is happening to her and is labeling her response to these symptoms as indicative of "going crazy." Her behavioral and problem-solving repertoire essentially does not work in the present context.

Our 4:00 p.m. patient, Sheila Kelly, 55, is in *long-term survivorship* from a nasopharyngeal cancer, for which radical surgery and full-head radiation therapy was provided more than 20 years ago. She had a remarkably good adjustment during survivorship, considering the extent of her cancer and its treatment. Now, the probable long-term effects of the treatment itself are burdening her with pain, fatigue, loss of mobility, a sense of rapid and premature aging, and an increasing restriction in daily activities. She is facing a decision about giving up work, which represents autonomy, financial security, and a source of social support and meaning. Compounding her concerns, she is receiving multiple and conflicting views about the nature of her pain, its causes, and its management. She recognizes that she has been blessed with long-term survival, but she also is disturbed by the fact that no one seems to understand the exact nature and impact of radiation therapy, more than 20 years post treatment. And this leads her to become angry and demoralized when she senses that members of the care team either do not accept her complaints as valid or understand what to do about her pain and fatigue. Sheila has displayed remarkable grit and tenacity in the more than 20 years since she was diagnosed with cancer. She continued to work, until very recently, in a physically demanding occupation, operating heavy equipment at a manufacturing plant. She has exercised and maintained a healthy diet. She pays careful attention to her medical needs and manages the demands of daily life to family and work with diligence and effectiveness. She is now becoming discouraged and depressed in the face of increasing pain and disability, which she fears will only have a downward course, until she fears ending up in a wheelchair. Her predictions of her life course may well be accurate; a potentially tragic outcome related to the long-term effects of her cancer and the radiation therapy she received as a treatment. Helping her stave off further disability, manage the pain more effectively, and accepting and finding a new balance between engagement and rest will be a part of the treatment plan to be developed in subsequent chapters.

Chapter Summary

Efforts to organize the response to cancer diagnosis, treatment, survivorship, and end-of-life processes were briefly reviewed. Empirically supported therapies including Cognitive Behavior Therapy and Problem-Solving Therapy have identified common adjustment and problem-solving strategies that impede or enhance adaptation to cancer. These were reviewed. Common psychological and physical challenges, by phase of treatment and recovery, were also reviewed. These include depression, anxiety, cognitive impairment, fatigue, and pain. The use of screening tools, in identifying these challenges was reviewed, in addition to the contexts and problem areas in which they arise.

Key Points

1. It is important to identify the adjustment and problem-solving orientations and style that each patient brings to the experience of having cancer.
2. Two evidence-based therapies, CBT and PST, are available to draw upon in understanding patient adjustment and problem-solving orientations and styles.
3. Avoidant and hopelessness-based problem solving contribute to poorer treatment adherence and poorer psychosocial outcomes.
4. Patients with cancer are at a heightened risk of both depression and anxiety disorders.
5. Sub-syndromal depression and anxiety problems need to be addressed, as they are both relatively common and affect adaptation to cancer.
6. The use of visual analog scales, to pinpoint distress, is both pragmatically useful and non-stigmatizing in nature.
7. Pinpointing distress, psychosocial problems, and physical problems allows for their incorporation into a case formulation to guide therapy.

8. Heuristic models were identified that allow the oncology team to pinpoint challenges and difficulties that patients may experience at various phases of care, from the initial diagnosis, to the treatment phase, to various stages of survivorship, to recurrence, and end-of-life status.

9. Knowledge derived from longitudinal and cross-sectional research on adaptation to cancer can allow the clinician to pinpoint the psychological and physical processes that are affecting adaptation, positively and negatively, and to target those for intervention.

Two
Re-Visioning Cognitive Behavior Therapy for Cancer Patients

There is an old saying that engineers want to know *how* something works, while scientists want to know *why* something works. Most of us who do clinical work understandably want to know the tools and techniques required to do effective therapy. We want to know *how* something works, and we may not steep ourselves in the *why*. Yet knowing something about the science and the theories behind tools and techniques is vital. Without this knowledge, the clinician is hampered, especially in those tough, but frequent, clinical moments when we are in new ground, and in which we must invent. This chapter addresses some of the important scientific and theoretical developments emerging in CBT over the past 20 years. These developments are organized into eight principles, which will guide therapy for the remainder of the book. If the reader prefers, feel free to skip to the summary and key points which appear at the end of this chapter. You can then return to this chapter later if you wish. Keep in mind that a general model, for a "re-visioned" Cognitive Behavior Therapy, is provided here. Specific applications of the model, for psycho-oncology, are detailed in the clinical chapters that follow. Those chapters will demonstrate the practical applications of every key point covered in this chapter.

Aaron T. Beck's Cognitive Therapy is among the most widely researched and disseminated form of Cognitive Behavior Therapy in the world. CBT has already established itself as a useful treatment for depression and anxiety with cancer and other medical patients (Antoni, 2003; Moorey & Greer, 2012; Levin et al. 2013, Levin, White, Bialer et al., 2013), as has a related form of CBT, Problem-Solving Therapy (Nezu et al., 1999; Nezu et al., 2012). Yet over the past 20 years, there have been important new research findings on cognition and human information processing, mindfulness, acceptance, emotion regulation, human change processes, and evolutionary biology and psychology. These findings have led to controversies in the field as well as the potential for significant advances in our understanding of human suffering and its alleviation. This chapter will briefly summarize those findings, and provide a list of principles, drawn from those findings, that will serve as the basis for a model of CBT for cancer patients. These, in turn, will allow us to create effective case conceptualizations and treatment strategies.

Cognitive Behavior Therapy is perhaps best understood as a family of therapies, all sharing a common commitment to science (Hofmann, 2012). As in any family, there is unity at times, discord at others. There can be competition, differing agendas, and seemingly irreconcilable points of view. The shared commitment to science sets the stage for creating testable hypotheses about mechanism and about treatment outcomes. The internecine battles in the field will likely ultimately be settled by scientific methods. So we can, in the meantime, learn from one another and be more lighthearted about our differences. Otherwise, we fall prey to the tendency that Freud described, which he termed "the narcissism of small differences" (Freud, 1958, p. 305).

Cognitive behavioral therapies share a commitment to understanding the complex relationship among cognition, emotion, behavior, and person-environment interaction. Similarly, they tend to focus on the present, socialize patients to a specific conceptualization of their difficulties, create goals and agendas for each session, and emphasize a transfer of learning to the daily environment via homework (Leahy, 2016). But the most widely known and researched of these therapies, Beck's CBT, Acceptance and Commitment Therapy (ACT), Dialectical Behavior Therapy (DBT), Metacognitive Therapy (MCT), Mindfulness-Based Cognitive Therapy (MBCT) and, more recently, Compassion Focused Therapy (CFT), all have slightly differing assumptions, philosophies, scientific paradigms, and clinical models. This book is written in the spirit of pulling together elements of various models, organized around a CBT case conceptualization (Kuyken et al., 2009; Persons, 2008; Wills & Sanders, 2013; Bennett-Levy et al., 2015, Wills, 2015), and with a theoretical framework that allows for a coherent integration of elements in each model. It seems that the time is right for this effort, both within the field of CBT and in the treatment of cancer patients. First, in treating cancer, medical advances are leading to new, targeted treatments, sometimes based on genetic testing, and on bolstering patient immune functioning. Advances in CBT have helped us to understand and to target the core processes that maintain human psychological suffering in ways that we did not understand perhaps 20 years ago. Combining the advances not only of medical science and technology, but also of psychological science, and the technologies available in CBT, allows us to provide the maximum help possible to the cancer patients we serve.

Steve Hayes (2015), a co-founder of Acceptance and Commitment Therapy wrote:

> The way I usually say it is there is a clearing in the woods and several pathways to it. The pathway we forged was based on our take on behavior analysis

and mostly we had to hack through jungle to make the path . . . we had little intention of arriving at that particular clearing. . . . They all call it different things and some of the corners are a little different than others . . . but it's all one big field.

(Hayes, 2015, ACBS listserv)

My own path to this "clearing in the woods" is reflected in this book. It is rooted in Beck's Cognitive Therapy and influenced by new models emerging in the field. In that clearing, Western science has met ancient meditative and contemplative traditions. CBT and the science on which it is built have arrived at new understandings of cognition and the context in which humans think and use language. We have a richer understanding of human change processes. We can make informed speculation about key components in how to foster change. We have a better understanding of the learning processes that make us unique as a species. We also better understand how the same processes which create vast adaptive advantages for humans, over other species, can go awry. We can be left vulnerable to the tyranny of language gone awry, to biases in thinking, to seemingly out-of-control mental and behavioral processes, and engagement in inflexible, rule-dominated behavior that damages lives, others and ours, and impairs our ability to see clearly, accept inevitable pain, and choose wisely how to meet both the challenges and the opportunities of daily life.

The hopeful news is that here in this clearing there are new ways to understand how we get stuck and how to become more free. If, as Siddhartha Mukherjee has suggested, we need to change and adapt and use every bit of our inventiveness to help those with cancer, the knowledge now available in CBT is likely to help. This effort preserves what I see as the heart of Beck's Cognitive Behavior Therapy, while taking into account those new developments in the field that have occurred in the 40 years since the model's creation.

This next section lays out the eight key organizing principles that will serve as the underpinning for the case conceptualizations and interventions with cancer patients used in this book. The theory and science behind these principles will be reviewed. Understanding these principles, and the science and theory behind them, is central to being able to respond effectively to the many unanticipated things that occur in our therapy sessions. When we face situations for which no manual has prepared us, we need to invent. Knowing a good theory, and knowing what's behind the theory, is a key to being able to invent in a disciplined way. It is what separates the master clinician from others. And it is to those who aspire to becoming master clinicians that this book is directed.

Let's now take a look at the eight key organizing principles, which form the bedrock of a re-visioned Cognitive Behavior Therapy for cancer patients. We will then take each in turn, and I will show how these principles relate to and build upon one another to create a robust therapeutic framework:

1. Normalizing human suffering;
2. Balancing, acceptance, mindfulness, and change processes;

3. A focus on transdiagnostic processes in psychological disorders;
4. Balancing cognitive and experiential interventions in CBT;
5. An increased focus on self-processes in therapy;
6. A more contextual model of human functioning;
7. A focus on strengths, resilience, and well-being;
8. The disciplined use of the therapist's self in fostering the treatment relationship.

Normalizing Human Suffering

The idea that pain is a ubiquitous part of human life is an ancient one, embedded in the world's wisdom and spiritual traditions. The Buddha's quest 2,500 years ago, for example, was rooted in his observation that pain is an inevitable part of a human life: we age, we become ill, we may suffer the effects of poverty and loss, we will all eventually die (Nhat Hanh, 2001). Rather than being a dismal and despairing philosophy, these insights allowed The Buddha to distinguish between pain and suffering and to become free of suffering, even when the inevitable pain within life occurs. As John Teasdale, a founder of Mindfulness-Based Cognitive Therapy observed: "The Buddha saw that unpleasant or uncomfortable physical sensations or emotional feelings are inherent in life. In themselves, they are not the problem" (Teasdale & Chaskalson, 2011a, p. 91). It is thus the way we relate to those sensations, feelings, and thoughts that creates suffering, rather than "normal" pain.

To face losing everything, to face a life that is not going according to our own personal plan, can be disillusioning, crushing, terrifying. Regardless of whether they meet criteria for *DSM-5* depressive and/or anxiety disorders, it is important for our patients to know that they are neither defective nor alone. As one cancer patient put it, upon his referral to a psychologist: "It's one thing to have cancer. But now my doctor thinks I am also crazy." The idea that emotional and physical pain is part of the human condition imparts a realistic dignity and levels the playing field between therapist and patient: we are truly all in this together.

This perspective is based on not only ancient wisdom, but also newer scientific and clinical advances in the field of CBT. A broader view of distress recognizes that humans are like jugglers: we build repertoires of coping behaviors that are broad enough to meet the demands of an ever-changing environment. However, given factors such as temperament, history, social milieu, and one's coping repertoire, each of us has a number of stressors beyond which we may cease to be effective jugglers. When this happens, we can metaphorically drop some or all of the juggling pins we are trying to keep in the air. Cancer can add a number of new stressors that simply tax one's ability to cope.

Although Beck's Cognitive Therapy is a transdiagnostic model, it evolved primarily in the context of treating *DSM* disorders. Several new models of CBT have broadened, normalized, and de-stigmatized psychological pain and suffering even further.

Acceptance and Commitment Therapy (ACT) recognizes that human suffering is built on the human tendency to fall into language traps, which become entailed with patterns of avoidance, and with engagement in behavior patterns that pull us out of living a vital life (Hayes et al., 2012). Not content to provide yet another treatment for specific *DSM* disorders, ACT boldly set forth an agenda intended to provide a psychological account of human suffering. That account of suffering is rooted in the very heart of human language and is explained through a behavioral account of language, in the form of Relational Frame Theory (RFT) (Hayes et al., 2001; Ramnero & Toerneke, 2008; Toerneke, 2010). In addition, ACT restores a focus on self-processes (Hayes, 1984; Hayes, Villatte et al., 2011) to psychology in a way that hearkens back to the work of William James (1890).

Dialectical Behavior Therapy (DBT), which was developed for chronically suicidal or parasuicidal patients with borderline personality, also recognizes this distinction between pain and suffering. DBT also de-stigmatizes human pain and encourages people to do what works in order to have a life worth living, rather than remaining stuck in unworkable patterns, dictated by temperament, history, and, for lack of a better term, practice. Among the three pillars of DBT are dialectics, radical behaviorism, and adaptations of Buddhist mindfulness and other contemplative practices (Linehan, 1993a; Koerner, 2012; Linehan, 2015).

Finally, newer therapy models deepen CBT's roots in evolutionary biology and psychology. Beck recognized the evolutionary roots of fear and sadness. Each is a response to impending or actual loss or threat, which serve adaptive functions for humans. Each is capable of going awry, on the basis of the tendency to misappraise threats and/or underestimate or underutilize resources for managing threats. Newer CBT models have taken fresh steps linking the field to evolutionary thinking as well. Linehan has described the evolutionary functions of emotion and their connection to action urges. In addition, the fundamental need for validation by others, and the consequences of invalidating environments, link her work to evolutionary theory.

Paul Gilbert's work has addressed the evolutionary roots of human compassion, rooted deeply in the need for connection and safety (Gilbert, 2004; 2009a); Gilbert & Choden, 2014). Gilbert identified three biologically based types of primal emotion regulation systems. All serve evolutionary adaptive functions for survival: a threat protection system, a drive (resource-seeking) system, and a self-soothing system (Gilbert, 2009a). Hayes & Sandford wrote that social connection preceded language (Hayes & Sanford, 2014), supporting the notion that tribal and family connection often exerts a powerful influence on thought, emotion, and behavior of individuals and groups. The need to be connected to others is fundamental, and is a central concern in formulating cases, conceptualizing the treatment relationship, and fostering social problem solving in CBT. We will see that this connects with the focus on contextualism, described as follows.

Summary

A re-visioned CBT for cancer is non-stigmatizing and helps patients learn that their distress has a logic and a function in the context of facing cancer. By connecting our work to principles of evolutionary biology and psychology, we not only normalize the response to distress but also encourage patients to tap into our evolutionarily adaptive needs for safety, soothing, and contact in times of distress. In addition, by normalizing human suffering in the face of cancer, we set the stage for psychoeducation, for reframing one's illness and coping narratives, and for deepening the therapeutic relationship, thus linking normalizing to other organizing principles in this approach.

Balancing, Acceptance, Mindfulness, and Change Processes

Acceptance

There has been a tremendous growth of mindfulness and acceptance-based therapies over the past 20 years, and a detailed review of the literature is well beyond the scope of this chapter (Hayes et al., 2004; Herbert & Foreman, 2011). For our purposes, one impetus for the development of mindfulness and acceptance-based therapies has been the awareness that our CBT change technologies have limits. Our treatment effects are limited. Perhaps the early promise of CBT met a wall of clinical reality that we could not move. We cannot change all the things that our patients bring to us in therapy. In addition, we are often working with clinical problems for which change is not possible. This may include adaptation to medical illnesses as well as the struggle against many other unbendable realities.

For these and perhaps a number of other reasons, the first mindfulness-based treatment, Jon Kabat-Zinn's Mindfulness-Based Stress Reduction model (Kabat-Zinn, 2013) found fertile ground in which to grow. The model evolved in a department of medicine and for patients who had reached the limits of what Western medicine could help. When we cannot rid ourselves of an aversive experience— pain, cancer, our life histories, our hurtful emotions and memories—another door must open in order to reduce suffering. A paradoxical form of change occurs when we cease to resist inner experience and unchangeable inner and outer realities.

Acceptance involves making room for and even embracing what is, rather than fighting it in ways that are self-damaging. Our histories happened. Our medical problems are as they are. Physical pain may be present, as might be fatigue, for a long time, if not forever. Working with, rather than fighting, reality is a central part of the newer, acceptance-based therapies. This does not mean approving of the injustices, adversities, pain, or disease that life has visited upon us, just seeing it as it is, and working with it differently. Marsha Linehan has described acceptance as playing the hand of cards that life deals us, rather than folding our hand and leaving the game. Cancer can be in the hand of cards life deals us.

Dialectical Behavior Therapy (Linehan, 1993a,b; 2015) was perhaps the first CBT model to integrate mindfulness and acceptance into the core of cognitive behavioral work. DBT now has more empirical support for the treatment of suicidal and parasuicidal behavior in borderline personality disorder than any other therapy (Stoffers et al., 2012). Key features of the model with regard to acceptance include the following:

1. A recognition that Acceptance is as important in dealing with human suffering as is change. Radical Acceptance involves a commitment to deep, all-the-way acceptance of life as it is, including one's emotional and behavioral repertoire, one's life history, pain and disappointments, and of reality. That commitment recognizes that one may not Radically Accept all at once; it can be a step-by-step turning of the mind toward acceptance.
2. A practical adaptation of Buddhist and other contemplative psychologies, including a detailed technology of mindfulness and acceptance practices to complement DBT's change technology.
3. Like ACT, the use of contemplative and mindfulness practices are employed to help access and cultivate what Linehan has called Wise Mind, or compassionate and wise self-states that transcend the medical model on which *DSM* is based, making DBT as much a life way as it is a treatment tool.

Linehan has drawn on the work of contemplative psychologist Gerald May (1982), who contrasted a willing, open, and accepting stance toward life with one of willful resistance to life's realities. Willfulness can be exhausting. It can be implicated in the development and maintenance of unworkable coping strategies, as we will see in subsequent chapters (Wills & Sanders, 2013).

Acceptance and Commitment Therapy (ACT) fosters an openness to experience, including unpleasant and disturbing thoughts, images, body sensations, emotions, and memories, without resisting or avoiding them. From this open stance toward experience, one is freer to choose new ways of relating to experience and new ways of being in the world. ACT's emphasis on addressing experiential avoidance (EA) dovetails with the findings of Harvey et al. (2004) on experiential avoidance as a transdiagnostic factor in depression and anxiety. EA is a factor related to poorer psychological outcomes in cancer patients (Stanton et al., 2015), making it a potentially important assessment and treatment target when working with this population.

Beck, too, has recognized the importance of acceptance in treating anxiety disorders, though it was not as central a focus in treatment as were cognitive change strategies.

The importance of acceptance in Beck's Cognitive Therapy is evident in the A-W-A-R-E strategy (A. Beck & Emery, 1985; A. Beck & Dozois, 2011; D.A. Clark & Beck, 2012), an acronym for:

1. Accept anxiety, instead of fighting against anxiety;
2. Watch your anxiety, observing anxiety in a non-judgmental manner;
3. Act with anxiety;

4. Repeat steps 1–3 as needed;
5. Expect the best, as you set the goal of strengthening your ability to tolerate anxiety.

British CBT models, too, emphasize an open, accepting posture toward anxiety, with treatment involving the willingness to face fear situations without use of neutralizing or avoidance strategies called safety behaviors (Bennett-Levy et al., 2004; Westbrook et al., 2012). Hofmann (2012) addressed the role of acceptance in Modern CBT and wisely described the way in which, for pain, we help remove the pain that can be changed, while fostering acceptance where pain removal or reduction is not currently possible. Levin et al. (2013), Levin, White, Bialer et al. (2013), and Moorey and Greer (2012) briefly touched on acceptance in their accounts of CBT for cancer patients. Yet it must be said that all the newer CBT therapies make acceptance *a central focus of their models*. In adapting CBT for work with cancer patients, we are well advised to include acceptance work in our assessment, our treatment formulations, and our intervention strategies.

Mindfulness

A full description of the literature on mindfulness, too, is well beyond the scope of this book (Wells, 2009; Grabovac et al., 2011; Herbert & Foreman, 2011; Teasdale & Chaskalson, 2011 a,b; Segal et al., 2013; Baer, 2014; Langer, 2014; Williams, M. et al., 2015). While there are considerable controversies regarding even the definition of mindfulness, mindfulness is at heart a way of relating to experience (Williams, M. et al., 2015). The British parliamentary report *Mindful Nation UK* defined mindfulness as "paying attention to what's happening in the present moment in the mind, body and external environment, with an attitude of curiosity and kindness" (MAPPG, October, 2015, p. 8). It is a set of methods for directing attention and cultivating the capacity to stay with experience, without fleeing from it, and to do so while observing experience with lightheartedness, compassion, and without entanglement in judgments. It is a mode of functioning that is experiential, rather than one that lends itself to talking about mindfulness.

Mindfulness is a component of ACT as well as a core of DBT, MCT, and MBCT. Lau and McMain (2005) described strategies for integrating acceptance and mindfulness into CBT as well. Each model defines mindfulness somewhat differently, and again, the reader is directed to the primary readings of each model to become acquainted in depth with how mindfulness is being incorporated into CBT. For our purposes, the most influential therapies that incorporate mindfulness are Mindfulness-Based Cognitive Therapy (MBCT), Dialectical Behavior Therapy (DBT) and Acceptance and Commitment Therapy (ACT). These are chosen because each has developed detailed and specific practices that readily translate into work with cancer patients.

Mindfulness-Based Cognitive Therapy (MBCT) blends Mindfulness-Based Stress Reduction, the mindfulness program developed by Jon Kabat-Zinn (2013) at the University of Massachusetts, with a scientific account of cognitive therapy and human information processing for depression relapse (Segal et al., 2001; 2013; Crane, 2009; Williams, M. et al., 2015). Originally developed as a relapse prevention treatment, MBCT is currently being studied as a means of treating acute depression as well (Baer & Walsh, 2016). MBCT is a structured, group-administered treatment that teaches a variety of meditative techniques, which the patient is expected to practice for up to 45 minutes a day, during the course of the entire 8-week program. Recognizing that rumination is a central component in depression relapse, linked to what Teasdale described as a "differential activation hypothesis" (Lau et al., 2004), MBCT attempts to break the link between depressed or sad mood, activation of depressive memories, and rumination. In addition to providing an intensive course in a wide variety of mindfulness practices, MBCT also teaches patients about their vulnerabilities to relapse, in the form of their personal relapse signature, and how to utilize their mindfulness training to prevent dropping back into depression.

Emerging data from recent studies suggest the following regarding vulnerability to depression relapse and the mechanisms of change in MBCT. First, people with three or more prior episodes of depression respond better to MBCT. The findings appear to be explained on the basis of two things. First, such patients seem to have an earlier onset of depression. Second, and perhaps more important, these patients have a higher rate of early childhood adverse experiences, especially including abuse and neglect (Segal et al., 2013; Williams, M. et al., 2015). A higher rate of adverse childhood experiences (ACE) is also found in other poor health outcomes and suggests that this finding in MBCT may be highly germane in treating psychologically vulnerable cancer patients (Corso et al., 2008; Anda et al., 2010; Brown et al., 2010).

The mechanisms by which MBCT achieves its results are posited to include the following:

1. An increase in the capacity for mindfulness (Segal, Williams, and Teasdale's "being mode");
2. A reduction in emotional and behavioral reactivity to depressive thoughts, memories, images, and emotions;
3. Dampened reactivity to depressive content including suicidal ideation, even if the frequency of such content does not necessarily decline;
4. Reduced engagement in the toxic process of rumination;
5. An increase in self-compassion, perhaps modeled by the instructor.

An important criticism of MBCT is that it may be top-heavy with a focus on mindfulness and underweighted in the use of the behavioral and cognitive behavioral technologies (Zettle, 2007).

DBT, in contrast, offers a balance of mindfulness and change technologies, combining as it does the wisdom of contemplative traditions with the technologies available in cognitive behavior therapy. DBT trains people in a secular adaptation of Buddhist psychology, to build attentional abilities as well as the ability to simply describe moment-to-moment experience without either falling prey to the tendency of the mind to confuse fact with judgment or to impulsively and blindly react to thoughts and emotions. DBT, for a variety of reasons, does not employ meditation, as MBCT does. Rather, both ACT and DBT foster the ability to enter present moment experiences, including via five-senses exercises, guided imagery, and mindfulness of breath. These models are practical and are focused on helping people pause, notice experience, and choose strategies to manage distress skillfully. Mindfulness and acceptance practices in DBT are intended to help patients access and cultivate what Linehan has called Wise Mind, or compassionate and wise self-states that transcend the medical model on which *DSM* is based, making DBT as much a life way as it is a treatment tool. Similarly, ACT trains the kind of perspective-taking skills that foster access to wise and compassionate self-states, making ACT, too, as much a life way as it is a therapy.

Two group administered mindfulness-based approaches to cancer treatment draw on mindfulness training, and both evolved from Jon Kabat-Zinn's Mindfulness-Based Stress Reduction (MBSR) (Kabat-Zinn, 2013). Carlson and Speca (2010) and Speca et al. (2000) developed Mindfulness-Based Cancer Recovery, which has developed a base of empirical support. Mindfulness-Based Cognitive Therapy influenced the development of Bartley's Mindfulness-Based Cognitive Therapy for Cancer (Bartley, 2012). Newer Cognitive Behavior Therapies, especially Acceptance and Commitment Therapy (ACT) have begun to demonstrate efficacy in treating cancer patients, as well (Feros et al., 2013; Rost et al., 2012; Williams et al., 2015; Arch & Mitchell, 2016;).

It is intuitively obvious how and why an acceptance focus is of importance in treating cancer patients, although skillfully fostering acceptance without hectoring the patient is required. Mindfulness in a variety of forms can be employed in both individual and group treatments, to build attentional processes and to help patients attune to non-cancer present moment processes via sensory awareness. We will focus in subsequent chapters on how to respectfully and effectively encourage acceptance moves in individual and couple therapy sessions and how acceptance can be carried forth into the patient's daily life. Similarly, how, when, and why to include mindfulness work in cancer treatment will be explored. Mindfulness and acceptance are often modeled by the therapist in such encounters, and strategies to promote a present-centered focus in the therapy relationship (Wilson & DuFrene, 2009) will be described, as will examples of utilizing mindfulness practices and skills to achieve a wide variety of therapeutic purposes. Those will be described, with ample clinical examples and applications, in subsequent chapters.

Summary

Mindfulness with cancer patients serves to help patients pause, attend, notice, choose, and act. It is a means of directing attention and awareness, intentionally and with compassion, while noticing the flow of experience as it occurs in the context of daily life. Then, the door to choice is opened. For purposes of this model, mindfulness and skillful action are tightly linked. Evan Thompson, a philosopher and neuroscientist, stated that mindfulness "is not a neural network, but how you live your life in the world" (Heuman, 2014). Mindfulness thus links to other principles in this book, by emphasizing its foundational role in supporting wise action for self-soothing, active engagement in problem solving, and acceptance of what is, as a condition of working with the givens of one's life, with wisdom and effectiveness. Our focus will be on mindfulness practices that can be used to good effect in briefer, focused individual and couples therapy.

A Focus on Transdiagnostic Processes in Psychological Disorders

The primary model used to explain human suffering in the United States is, broadly, a medical one, built on and employing the *Diagnostic and Statistical Manual of the American Psychiatric Association* (American Psychiatric Association, 2013). Increasingly, the field of CBT has searched for transdiagnostic psychological factors to understand clinical disorders, especially depression and anxiety disorders (Barlow et al., 2004).

Understanding these processes thus advances the effort to link theory, science, and clinical practice in CBT.

Multiple streams of research have demonstrated the human tendency for cognitive biases. Beck's Cognitive Therapy was built on this premise (A. Beck & Dozois, 2011; A. Beck & Haigh, 2014). There is now ample evidence to validate at least some of Beck's early observations about cognitive biases.

A landmark book, *Cognitive Behavioural Processes Across Psychological Disorders* by Harvey et al. (2004), reviewed evidence and concluded that there is strong empirical support for the following transdiagnostic processes in both depression and anxiety disorders, which are the most common presenting problems in cancer patients, and which form the clinical focus of this book:

1. *Selective attention*, which is the tendency for human attention to be biased toward specific, concern-related outer and inner stimuli and to sources of safety.
2. *Memory biases*, both as explicit selective memory and recurrent memory. The mind, as it were, involuntarily selects memory that is biased in the direction of specific concerns, including loss, diminishment, and threat. And the mind can at times experience recurrent, intrusive, disturbing, and/or maladaptive memory that is both repetitive and seemingly involuntary.
3. *Reasoning biases*, including biased interpretation of ambiguous stimuli, biased inferences about causal outcomes in life, and a variety of biased

expectancies and heuristics, including the tendency to seek data that confirm one's pre-existing beliefs. Note that these biases broadly confirm Beck's own clinically derived observations of "cognitive errors."

4. *Rumination and worry*, which impair effective problem solving, with rumination being more focused on themes of loss and a damaged and diminished sense of self, and worry tending to involve a focus on imagined future threats and intolerance of uncertainty.

5. *Positive and negative metacognitive beliefs*, which are essentially beliefs about the mental operating system, seen as either dangerously out of control, or viewing worry and rumination as necessary, functional strategies.

6. The use of *avoidance and safety behaviors*, which involves avoidance of both inner and outer threats, real and imagined, in ways that dampen effective problem solving and more accurate, flexible appraisals of threat.

Nobel laureate and cognitive psychologist Daniel Kahneman (2011) provided independent lines of research that support Harvey et al.'s conclusions with regard to the human tendency toward cognitive biases. Beck's early model emphasized addressing these biases in cognitive content via evidence testing and creating new alternative beliefs. Yet cognitive therapy actually attempts to modify both form and function of thoughts, depending upon the circumstances (A. Beck & Dozois, 2011).

More recent developments in CBT, particularly in Metacognitive Therapy (MCT), have created new ways of conceptualizing and intervening in cognitive *processes* that go awry, chiefly in the form of seemingly out-of-control worry and rumination (Wells, 2000; 2009). A recent study has suggested that specific types of worry and avoidance behaviors are related to symptoms of anxiety, depression, and PTSD in cancer patients (Cook et al., 2015). In subsequent chapters, I will provide strategies for dealing with biases in cognitive content as well as the processes of runaway worry and rumination.

Summary

Pinpointing relevant transdiagnostic processes in our case formulations allows us to create case formulations that guide treatment and to target those processes with carefully selected interventions. In dealing with the diagnosis and treatment of cancer, patients can have cognitive biases: "I'm as good as dead," "My life as I've lived it is over," "I can't handle this." In addition, maladaptive cognitive processes can easily occur in cancer patients, chiefly through unproductive forms of worry and rumination. CBT can target threat estimates, foster more adaptive appraisals of one's ability to manage cancer, and decrease engagement in destructive forms of worry and rumination.

Balancing Cognitive and Experiential Interventions in CBT

Beck's CBT has always believed in the power of the mind to use rationality and logic to heal oneself. Beck's CBT is predicated on the assumption that it is the meaning of events that most influences one's reactions to events (A. Beck & Dozois, 2011; A. Beck & Haigh, 2014). Yet meaning is not always encoded in purely verbal ways. CBT has always recognized the centrality of emotionally encoded meaning, not just the more rational modes of information processing (Bennett-Levy et al., 2004; Leahy et al., 2011; Wills & Sanders, 2013; Wills, 2015). New developments in the field allow us to better understand the complexity of human information processing. We think not only in words but also in emotionally laden images and metaphor. We want interventions that address both the head and the heart and that speak to the emotional core of being human. These target the more rational, verbal modes of information processing as well as the more emotionally laden and less frankly verbally encoded levels of meaning.

At heart, Beck's early methods involved training patients to frame their beliefs in words, and to test those beliefs, in order to determine for themselves whether systematic biases or cognitive errors were impairing their functioning. We have already seen, in the previous section on transdiagnostic factors, that all humans are prone to systematic cognitive errors. Beck's clinical observations led to a cognitive specificity model, in which characteristic patterns of bias show up in specific disorders. From those general patterns, a more idiographic model, unique to the individual, is created as part of our case formulation for each patient. In the case of depression, these errors tend to involve misappraisals of self, world, and future, the "cognitive triad" of depression (A. Beck & Rush, 1979). In the case of anxiety disorders, Beck's model addresses the tendency of anxious patients to overestimate threat magnitude and probability, while underestimating one's ability to manage actual threat effectively (A. Beck & Emery, 1985).

In addition to the more verbally encoded and easily accessible automatic thoughts, Beck has posited that cognition is layered, such that the most accessible level of information processing takes the form of what he called automatic thoughts. Much work in CBT takes place at the level of addressing automatic thoughts. Indeed, for many of the *DSM* Axis I disorders, work at this level, and the level of rules and assumptions, is often sufficient to successfully complete therapy. Yet Beck has recognized that more developmentally embedded, emotionally encoded meaning, in the form of "core beliefs," drove human functioning as well. Work in the area of core beliefs began with depression (A. Beck & Rush, 1979) and became more central in CBT for personality disorders (A. Beck et al., 2006). The existence and nature of core beliefs has received less empirical support than automatic thoughts. And, as a result, case formulations that rely on increasingly inferential data decline in reliability across raters (Kuyken et al., 2009).

In addition, Beck has described an intermediate layer of cognition, which consists of rules and silent assumptions. Rules are ubiquitous in daily life and serve as a shorthand for engaged action and for making sense of the world. They may derive from rules observed implicitly or explicitly in one's family of origin or culture. They may also be almost entirely idiosyncratic and arbitrary to the individual. Inflexible and maladaptive rules may lead to suffering, to oneself and possibly to others (Beck, 2011a). Getting a sense of life as rule governed and fair. As one patient put it, "I have always taken care of myself with a good diet, no smoking, and exercise. I wasn't supposed to get lung cancer."

For a more behavioral account of rules, Hayes was able to demonstrate that rule-governed behavior, while serving a clear evolutionarily adaptive function, can also impair effective human living (Hayes et al., 1986). A rat in an operant chamber will have to go through many trials to learn that when a certain colored light is on it must push the right lever to get food and when another light is on it must push the left lever to get food. Humans can learn a rule, verbally (push right when red light on and left when green). They don't need to go through a potentially longer process of trial and error. But, when the contingency changes, for example if the lights are now reversed in terms of which lever they signal, humans may persist with the rule even though food is not being produced, whereas a rat will figure out after a few trials that the contingency changed.

Thus, rules serve the function of creating an economy of learning. But the lowered sensitivity to changing environmental conditions can pose problems for humans. Humans may be the only creature on the planet that will follow verbally mediated rules, even when they don't work. Human language can thus actually pull people out of the ability to accurately and flexibly assess and respond to the changing contingencies of the environment. Inflexible and maladaptive rules can be implicated in non-acceptance and in the persistence of coping strategies that impede effective coping with cancer's challenges. To make this practical and useful for understanding our cancer patients, consider the following: a patient lives by a rule that demands peak performance, even when one is exhausted and in pain, following surgery, chemotherapy, and/or radiation. Efforts to live by this rule may be a maladaptive setup for suffering. Persisting in following the rule "If I don't do everything expected of me, I'm a failure," will likely prove unworkable and out of touch with current realities. Instead, flexibility in adapting to the limitations imposed by cancer and cancer therapy is required. When contingencies change, rules must be flexibly adapted to meet those changes. Rules for living that served one well before cancer may not work in the present. This emphasis on cognitive biases, rules, and assumptions links with our principles involving acceptance and change.

Controversies in dealing with automatic thoughts and rules: I want to briefly address a key controversy that has arisen in the field, because it will be germane to our treatment efforts here. Challenges to cognitive techniques began to arise in a newly energized behaviorism, beginning in the 1980s and accelerating in the late 1990s (Jacobson et al., 1996; Martell et al., 2001; Dimidjian et al., 2006; Martell et al., 2010). At heart, Jacobson and associates have demonstrated that it is possible to effectively treat depression without using CBT's cognitive restructuring techniques. Other writers have questioned the scientific foundation of cognitive therapy's emphasis on testing and modifying thoughts (Longmore & Worrell, 2007). ACT, too, has challenged the use of Beckian rationalist techniques, on both scientific and philosophical grounds (Hayes, Villatte et al., 2011). ACT not only eschews Beckian techniques as unnecessary but also at times suggests that such techniques are iatrogenic (Zettle, 2016), to which Keefe and DeRubeis (2016) responded, "Given the robust literature of controlled experiments establishing the therapeutic efficacy of CBT for depression, a claim that to challenge thoughts (a core technique of CBTs) is *universally* iatrogenic is difficult to sustain and would require clear empirical confirmation" (p. 250). In a critique somewhat similar to ACT's, Wells noted that "the MCT therapist does not focus on the content of beliefs, except those at the metacognitive level" (Wells & Fisher, 2016b, p. 163). In response, Keefe and DeRubeis (2016) questioned whether metacognition actually represents another level of cognition.

I would suggest that while the purported mechanisms of change in CBT remain an elusive and controversial topic, it is wise to accept the findings articulated by Teasdale et al. (1995). To wit: Beckian cognitive interventions, and perhaps all cognitive interventions, work by changing one's relationship to thoughts, rather than by ridding one of presumed maladaptive thoughts, as a precondition for change. This distinction is somewhat subtle but appears to be scientifically and theoretically sound. In effect, then, while Beck's CBT may be uniquely positioned to help people identify and correct cognitive biases, it does so not by stopping the maladaptive thoughts as a precondition for change, but by helping people access more flexible and pragmatically functional alternative ways of viewing oneself and one's circumstances. Given the fact that depressed and anxious cancer patients may not show evidence of the cognitive distortions Beck identified, it is important to have other means of addressing psychological suffering, including a more experiential focus.

ACT therapists have created a rich array of experiential interventions to help people spring free of the traps of language and experiential avoidance that are a hallmark of inflexible responding to life (Hayes, Villatte et al., 2011; Stoddard & Afari, 2014). These interventions differ in many ways from standard Beckian techniques, yet also help promote the ends specified by Teasdale: a changed relationship to one's thoughts, one which allows more flexible responding. The model employed here, then, draws on ACT's experiential work, while recognizing and retaining Beckian CBT strategies for dealing with cognitive biases, especially in the not infrequent situations when such biases can rapidly be addressed by such interventions. The use of these techniques will be seen as compatible with the emphasis in ACT on psychological flexibility. We will deal with guidelines for choosing intervention strategies in subsequent clinical chapters.

When logic fails: Words and logic may fail to adequately pierce the long-standing, emotionally laden material of human suffering (Gilbert, 2009a, 2010; Hayes,Villatte et al., 2011; Wills & Sanders, 2013), as Beck, too, understood (A. Beck & Dozois, 2011). Frequently, our patients notice a split between what the head experiences and what the gut experiences, and they are in such cases quite different. This is a common finding in our consultation rooms: the patient notes that in the therapy session, she knows that her heart palpitations are harmless, but in the darkness of her home, in the middle of the night, she fears that she is dying of brain metastases, despite repeated scans to the contrary.

The science and theories that may explain *why* words and logic can fail us may lie in the tendency of humans to process information in multiple levels or modes, some more emotionally laden and processed with images and body sensations, while other modes are more verbally mediated and hence subject to verbal examination, refutation, and the creation of believable and workable alternatives. It is when our modes of processing are in conflict, between the head and the heart, between reason and emotion, that problems may arise. This awareness, too, is embedded in ancient wisdom and forms the bedrock for many theories of psychotherapy, from psychoanalysis to current CBT models. It is also a subject of study by researchers in other areas of psychology, including those affiliated with Positive Psychology (Haidt, 2006).

Thus, work with imagery, metaphor, and experiential interventions all have come increasingly into play in CBT, particularly within the British CBT community (Gilbert, 2009a; 2010; 2014; Stott et al., 2010; Hackmann et al., 2011; Westbrook et al., 2012; Wills & Sanders, 2013). There is evidence that the use of Behavioral Experiments in CBT, rather than reliance on Thought Records, produces more rapid cognitive change, and that beliefs about self and others generalized more effectively with Behavioral Experiments as well (McManus et al., 2011). This entire palette of interventions is available within the CBT tradition, in addition to mindfulness and self-process work. And within the ACT tradition, a large and fascinating array of powerful experiential exercises exist, drawing from a wide tradition of therapies, and organized around the scientific and theoretical core of the ACT model (Hayes et al, 2012; Stoddard & Afari, 2014).

Perhaps the best way to describe the aim of many of our cognitive and experiential strategies is the achieving of "metacognitive awareness" (Williams, M. et al., 2015). This involves the ability to observe and notice inner events as mental events, rather than as facts, as though one were literally standing behind a waterfall, watching the water falling, rather than being in the stream of water itself (Segal et al., 2001). Metacognitive awareness is one doorway into a place of choice, about how to relate to one's beliefs, rules, and assumptions as well as one's emotional experiences and physical sensations. And with this capacity for choice comes the ability to respond with flexibility, in line with one's intentions for addressing the demands and opportunities of the moment.

Finally, it is possible to influence both emotion and cognition through movement, posture, and through other sensory experiences. Linehan's (2015) use of a technique called "willing hands and half smile" is an example. Bennett-Levy et al. (2015) incorporated movement and posture into their Self-Practice/ Self-Reflection model. They drew on the innovative work of Korrelboom, whose COMET model (**CO**mpetitive **ME**mory Training) utilizes posture, music, and movement to help create self-states and accessible memory structures for people with self-esteem problems and depression (Ekkers et al., 2011; Korrelboom et al., 2012). Another influence on both Bennett-Levy and Korrelboom is the work of Brewin (2006), who developed a retrieval competition model of memory, which involves building self-states that are stored in memory and can compete successfully with older, less adaptive memory structures, activated in depressive and anxiety disorders, or in personality disorders.

Summary

Working with cancer patients demands the use of the full range of techniques and perspectives available in CBT for addressing cognition, emotion, and behavior patterns: assessing the content of thoughts for their accuracy and/or function; pinpointing cognitive biases; helping people unplug from toxic cognitive processes, such as worry and rumination; using experiential exercises to produce emotionally compelling change; working with imagery and metaphor; and utilizing body and posture work to not only downregulate emotional turbulence when warranted but also to help build new ways of being. As Williams noted, "the tricks that language can play on us are inexhaustible, so the methods we use to better understand these tricks and deal skillfully with them will also be inexhaustible" (McHugh & Stewart, 2012, pp. ix–x).

An Increased Focus on Self-Processes in Therapy

The notion of a self, or of various experiential self-states, was introduced into American psychology by William James (1890), who struggled with defining various aspects of self in terms of science versus metaphysics. Though intrigued by various spiritual, religious, and trance states, he leaned more in the direction of an empirical science and concluded his speculations about self by famously declaring "thoughts themselves are the thinkers" (James, 1890).

The renewed interest in self-processes certainly has roots in the increasing influence of Buddhist psychology in the West. As a matter of pragmatics, and for the sake of focus, we will remain anchored in the terms "self-processes" and "self-states" as they are being articulated within the more empirical wing of psychology and neurosciences. The work of Steve Hayes has restored the scientific and clinical interest in self-processes to a place of prominence (Hayes, 1984; Hayes, Strosahl, & Wilson, 2012). Tying self-processes together with perspective-taking skills, Hayes eventually developed theories and techniques to help people cultivate these processes. Perspective taking involves the ability to experience distinctions between "me-here-now" and "me-there-then" as well as between "me" and "other". Perspective-taking skills are in other therapy models as well (Spivack et al., 1976; Bateman & Fonagy, 2012). Hayes, however, cast perspective-taking skills into a behavioral and experiential account of language. Variously called self-as-content, self-as-context, transcendent self, these self-states, or self-processes, can be trained and accessed using the ACT model (Hayes et al., 2012: McHugh & Stewart, 2012; Villatte et al., 2012). Wilson et al. (2012) noted that self, from a behavioral perspective, is not a noun; it is a verb, a set of behavioral repertoires. Selfing, if you will, is a process, not a noun or a thing. This process is experiential, subject to constant change, and is linked to how we deploy awareness (Thompson, 2015).

Teasdale's work, and the nature of MBCT, fostered our understanding that humans have multiple information processing modes, as he described in his paper on "three modes of mind" (Teasdale, 1993). Teasdale's work has lent itself to the notion that we are helping people access self-processes that can be both healing and freeing. Brewin (2006) described how the creation of competing memory structures can help build new cognitive, emotional, and behavioral repertoires, which become increasingly accessible to the person in situations where the older more automatic, and maladaptive pattern was more likely to have been invoked. Bennett-Levy et al. (2015) built on this foundation as well, in their work on training therapists to use self-practice and self-reflection methods to "build new ways of being." These models built on Beck's original ideas of "modes" (A. Beck, 1996; A. Beck & Haigh, 2014). As was often the case, Beck opened a door, though it fell to others to develop and flesh out a key idea.

Summary

For our purposes, the "self" is a complex set of processes, both verbal and experiential. Self-states, or states of being (Bennett-Levy et al., 2015), are not reducible to the automatic thoughts or other verbal products of awareness: they are states that include body sensations, emotion, imagery and memory, action propensities, and posture. Self-states can be accessed, cultivated, and sustained through interventions that address any of these relevant domains. Helping cancer patients access and build upon chosen self-states will be a feature of our clinical model. First, it dignifies our work, and it comports with our efforts to de-stigmatize psychological suffering. Second, it helps people capitalize on potential teaching moments that cancer might create (Stanton et al., 2015), by accessing and/or building wise, compassionate self-states. In addition, as we will see, one's very sense of self can be challenged and altered by cancer in ways that lead patients to experience a loss of self and meaning. We will focus in clinical chapters on strategies and techniques to help people access and build these processes, or states of being, in all phases of cancer: diagnosis, treatment, survivorship, and when facing death.

A More Contextual Model of Human Functioning

The debate between mechanistic and contextual accounts of causality is thousands of years old and is salient to an understanding of ecology, biological systems, psychology, and psychotherapy. The debate accelerated with the rise of

Cartesian-Newtonian science and the subsequent account provided by Systems Theory (Capra & Luisi, 2014).

This dialectic between mechanistic and contextual accounts in science and philosophy was pivotal in the development of the Family Therapy movement, beginning in the 1960s (Gehart, 2014). More recently, contextual accounts of language and behavior have arisen primarily within the more behavioral wing of the field, through ACT (Hayes et al., 1993; Hayes, Villatte et al., 2011). While here, too, a detailed account of this debate is beyond the scope of the chapter, a few comments are in order. Understanding and creating a more contextual account of human functioning will be central to our efforts to understand and help struggling cancer patients. Some of the eight organizing principles in this book have been subsumed under the term "contextualism" in newer CBT models. To wit: Herbert et al. (2016) described the distinguishing characteristics of contextual CBT as including a focus on the function of thoughts and subjective experiences, rather than the form or frequency of such events. Mindfulness and acceptance are, too, considered distinguishing features of contextual CBT approaches. They also note that contextual approaches are transdiagnostic in nature, integrative in nature, and tend to apply to issues of "spirituality, meaning, and sense of self."

The model of contextualism presented here draws not only on newer, contextual CBT approaches (Herbert et al., 2016) but also on contextual models that foster an understanding of the person's relationship to the ecosystems in which behavior is embedded.

In this sense, contextual principles involve helping people navigate their relationship to internal processes, such as thoughts, images, body sensations, memories, and emotions. In addition, a contextual focus helps the person navigate the ecosystems in which they are embedded to achieve security, soothing, support, and collaboration. These ecosystems include the interpersonal worlds, ranging from medical teams, families, and other social contexts of importance.

Thinking and experiencing takes place in a context or, more precisely, multiple contexts simultaneously and moment-by-moment. The thought "I have cancer, so it means I'm going to die" takes place in the context of one's history of illnesses, one's family history of illness, the story or narrative one has woven about self in adversity, and in the outer contexts of personal relationships to others, including the care team. Both inner and outer contexts influence human behavior, including cognition. How one deals with the thought "I can't handle this" depends not only upon the historical and current contexts, internal and outer, but also on the purpose or function of "I can't handle this." Function is found not just in examining the thought for its truth but also for examining what happens when one behaves as though the thought were true, that is, its function in one's life. And function can be assessed by looking at whether one's behavior (including cognition and overt behavior) works or doesn't work. In other words, does it produce an effect that is consistent with what matters to one in the moment?

More recently within the field of CBT, Hayes deepened the discussion of contextual versus more mechanistic accounts, with regards to language and change

(Hayes,Villatte et al., 2011). Hayes's work, in ACT and Relational Frame Theory, stated the claim that its account is rooted in Functional Contextualism, one of the many forms that contextualism can take (Hayes et al., 1993; Hayes, Villatte et al., 2011). This account is built on pragmatism, a behavioral account of language, and the idea that the truth value of a belief or of overt behaviors is to be found in its *functions*. And this leads to a foundational assumption in ACT, based on a variety of contextualism called Functional Contextualism: all behavior, internal and overt, can be understood in terms of whether it works in the context of supporting one's objectives, including living in accordance with one's cherished values. Detailed accounts of Functional Contextualism can be found elsewhere (Toerneke, 2010; Hayes et al., 2012; Hayes, Villatte et al., 2011). However, the pragmatic roots of this form of CBT bear similarities to William James (1890), for whom "the truth is what works" (Cormier, 2001). The arcane becomes practical.

So is this merely the latest dustup between cognitivists and behaviorists? And is it a form of trivial hairsplitting between tribal factions within the field? No and no. It is more than that. Indeed, Hayes noted,

> The real distinctions are not a behavioral account of cognition versus a cognitive account. The real distinctions are a contextual account versus a mechanistic account, a technical account versus a lay account, and a historical account versus a biological account.
>
> (Personal communication, May 1, 2015)

The most mechanistic version of CBT would suggest that thoughts cause emotions and behavior, and that in order to change emotions and behavior, we must first change our thoughts. Beck never embraced this type of mechanism, yet CBT did evolve more in the direction of a mechanistic than a contextual account of language and change. For example, the theory of how CBT works is described here and is taken from the Beck Institute for Cognitive Therapy website: "Cognitive behavior therapy helps people identify their distressing thoughts and evaluate how realistic the thoughts are. Then they learn to change their distorted thinking. When they think more realistically, they feel better." This is a more frankly mechanistic account, in which thoughts > emotions/behavior, and in which a precondition for changing emotions/behavior is to first change thoughts.

More nuanced perspectives on the relationship between cognitive and behavior change are increasingly appearing within the CBT camp (Bennett-Levy et al., 2004; Wills & Sanders, 2013; A. Beck & Haigh, 2014; Bennett-Levy et al., 2015; Wills, 2015). One key, for our purposes, is to recognize that change anywhere in the broad context in which behavior (cognition or overt behavior) occurs can influence all other parts of the system. Recall the statement by the neuroscientist and philosopher Evan Thompson (Heuman, 2014) that mindfulness and cognition are not just "a neural network, but how you live your life in the world." CBT increasingly recognizes that thinking, action, and environmental feedback are reciprocally interrelated. This is a form of contextualism. Hayes altered the contextual paradigm by arguing for a functional contextualism, in which behavior, including cognition, is understood in terms of its purpose or function.

Let's take a simple example: a 45-year old cancer patient has avoided follow-up monitoring for several years, because "I don't want to hear bad news," "I couldn't handle it if I learned my cancer is back," and "I can't stand being scared again." So in the context of avoiding bad news, avoiding hearing that cancer might have returned, and avoiding fear, it works to refuse monitoring, for years. However, what if the context and purpose of monitoring is about something else: "I want to be there for my kids. I want to protect my life and my family." Action chosen depends upon one's purpose. Quite frequently, contextual thinking in cancer work involves helping foster purposeful engagement in activities that including the demands of treatment as well as effectively engaging in the reciprocity of soothing, support, love, and care of one's family, friends, co-workers, spiritual communities, and care teams.

Summary

A more contextual CBT adopts a less mechanistic account of language and of the person's engagement with the world. The person's inner life, of private experiences, is viewed as in reciprocal relationship with the environmental contexts in which one is nested. Understanding the functions and purposes of behavior allows us to direct our efforts at change to those processes most likely to produce pragmatic results. Finally, it is wise to preserve a spirit of playfulness in our therapeutic use of mechanism and contextualism. There are times when playing with mechanism is wise and prudent, even for an avowed contextualist, and there are times when contextualism is the wise and prudent perspective. The issue is for what problems, when, and toward what ends.

A Focus on Strengths, Resilience, and Well-Being

A focus on strengths and resilience has long been a cornerstone of a number of family therapy approaches (Boszormenyi-Nagy & Krasner, 1986; Hargrave & Pfitzer, 2003; Walsh, 2006; Gehart, 2014). This emphasis on strengths in families has extended to work with medically ill patients (Rolland, 1990; McDaniel et al., 2013) and is an important area to include in working with cancer patients and their families. Positive Psychology has also arisen in response to the recognition that human strengths and well-being are legitimate and important foci for intervention (Seligman & Csikszentmilhayi, 2000; Seligman et al., 2005; Lyubomirsky, 2007; Seligman, 2011).

Although CBT began as a treatment whose intended function was the dampening or removal of clinical syndromes such as depression and anxiety disorders, CBT has begun to move toward an emphasis on strengths, resilience, meaning, values, and well-being. Padesky and Mooney (2012) described a 4-stage model, which incorporates patient strengths into the case conceptualization and treatment approach. Kuyken et al. (2009) built strengths into their overall CBT case conceptualization model for not only solving problems and treating clinical disorders but also promoting lifelong resilience. Bennett-Levy et al. (2015) utilized a strength-based approach, combined with newer theories and strategies in CBT to train therapists to use CBT to apply the model in their own lives. This work drew on Brewin (2006), Padesky and Mooney (2012), and others in a creative synthesis of traditional CBT techniques, strengths, values, posture, and body movement to create new ways of being.

ACT's focus on values makes it, too, a resilience and strength-based approach to human suffering (Dahl et al., 2009). And DBT's stated purpose of helping people have lives worth living does the same. Values and well-being are finding their way increasingly into therapy for cancer (Breitbart et al., 2010). The newer CBT and Positive Psychology models thus offer a renewed theoretical and scientific foundation for this work to proceed.

Many cancer patients who appear for our services may never have utilized, or needed, psychological therapies before. Their histories are often replete with strong adaptive resources, all of which are capable of being brought to bear on helping them manage the challenge of cancer. Drawing on the strengths-based focus of newer CBT models will likely resonate with many people, is non-stigmatizing, and brings the best of emerging perspectives on change, meaning, and well-being into the consulting room.

Summary

A focus on patient strengths and resources helps shift the focus from pathology toward a more normalizing stance on suffering. And it helps both therapist and patient(s) access the resources patients have employed at other times when life posed challenges, in the service of managing the difficulties of cancer.

The Disciplined Use of the Therapist's Self in Fostering the Treatment Relationship

Central to all CBT models, and indeed all therapy models, are the principles of genuine compassion and caring, which includes the ability to shift between maintaining a validating, emotionally supportive stance and a stance that fosters change (Norcross & Lambert, 2013). CBT for cancer patients is predicated on the therapist first understanding the patient, then seeking to help foster change.

Beck was trained initially as a psychoanalyst (Weishaar, 1993), and he brought with him into CBT a strong focus on the treatment relationship. Combining CBT with a Rogerian core, Beck recognized that a strong therapeutic relationship was essential for conducting effecting CBT. In fact, he noted in his 1979 depression manual, that "before one can be a good Cognitive Therapist, one must first be a good psychotherapist" (A. Beck & Rush, 1979, p. 23). And the treatment relationship formed the bedrock of being a good therapist. Indeed, the Cognitive Therapy Rating Scale (Young & Beck, 1980) has a number of items that address the nature and quality of the therapeutic relationship, as do newer measures of CBT adherence and competence.

Built into the model are key principles for building and managing the treatment relationship, central of which are the use of Guided Discovery and Socratic Questioning. Guided Discovery is a stance of collaboration in which the patient is invited to be a co-investigator and explorer, together with the therapist. The therapist demonstrates genuineness, warmth, and compassion, and employs a gentle and questioning style. The use of Socratic Questioning is intended to spark curiosity in the patient, as the therapist and patient work together to uncover the sometimes hidden meanings behind the patient's difficulties and to collaborate in their resolution. The therapist never lapses into lecturing or badgering the patient into changing his or her thinking, a point that is sometimes lost on critics of the model.

Leahy writes extensively about the therapeutic relationship, including how to manage the impasses that can occur in CBT (Leahy, 2001). In addressing how the therapist works with patients who are experiencing tragedy or suffering, he advised that we "weep for the plague, not just attempt to cure it" (p. 57). He wrote: "When we experience what seems awful and horrible in our lives, we often take solace in knowing that another person understands, or, at least, is attempting to understand, our pain" (Leahy, 2001, p. 58).

Linehan wrote a seminal chapter on validation, which details a disciplined and heartfelt approach to validation and the treatment relationship (Linehan, 1997). Validation strategies dovetail with Guided Discovery and Socratic Questioning, one deepening the other. I believe that they can be easily combined and that doing so adds power to each model, CBT and DBT. Together, they create a method for deeply entering the patient's experience, to explore the logic that may be maintaining the patient's suffering. In this process, when done well, the patient experiences a deep sense of being understood, and a shared formulation can be created. The patient comes to understand the logic of their responses to problematic situations, while a road map is created to find a path out of suffering. Linehan has described six levels of validation, which will be described in more detail in Chapter 3. We will explore in detail how to combine Guided Discovery and Socratic Questioning with validation strategies.

Finally, therapist self-practice, using the principles employed in this book, encourages the therapist to use the same principles and tools for problem solving and growth that our patients employ. Bennett-Levy et al. (2015) discussed the importance of therapist self-practice and self-reflection in CBT as a means of building a high level of skills. MBCT, ACT, and DBT all advocate therapist practice of the model as a means of building both skills and credibility with patients. Given the acuity of suffering in cancer patients, the use of the principles in this book, by the therapist, is also advised. Chapter 9 will address this issue in more detail. But treating cancer patients can pull powerfully from our own fears, including the fear of death. And burnout among therapists can be amplified when working with any patient population whose suffering can touch the therapist to the core.

Summary

Combining DBT validation strategies with Beckian Guided Discovery and Socratic Questioning creates the opportunity for the therapist to create therapeutic relationships that are caring, effective, and powerful, blending the therapist's self with the disciplined use of CBT technologies. These tools, when genuinely embodied by the therapist, help normalize the patient's distress and set the stage for the use of acceptance and change strategies.

Chapter Summary

Eight interrelated organizing principles were outlined. These principles allow for the creation of effective case conceptualizations and careful selection of interventions to target relevant processes. These eight organizing principles will be used to identify and intervene with cancer patients from the diagnosis and treatment phase through long-term survivorship or end-of-life work.

Key Points

1. CBT for cancer is a non-stigmatizing model, which normalizes distress in the context of the adaptive challenges posed by cancer.
2. CBT for cancer employs a stress-diathesis model, in which temperament, coping repertoires, and stress loads are among the key explanatory factors in depression and anxiety.
3. The systematic, disciplined use of the therapist "self" is a key component of CBT for cancer.
4. Mindfulness and acceptance are balanced with a use of change strategies in CBT for cancer.
5. CBT teaches cancer patients to become more astute observers of self and better functional analysts of occasions when they might become entrapped in patterns of coping that keep them stuck in suffering.
6. CBT for cancer draws on a transdiagnostic model, pinpointing psychological processes implicated in human suffering, and integrating them with the biological challenges that cancer patients face from the disease and its treatments.
7. Cognition includes not only verbally encoded material but also meaning that is encoded via imagery, metaphor, and implicit meaning derived from emotion and body sensations.

8. Cognitive *content*, cognitive *function*, and cognitive *processes* (worry and rumination) are treatment targets that may require different conceptualizations and interventions from one another.

9. CBT draws on techniques that address verbally encoded meaning as well as more experiential techniques to address more emotionally encoded meaning, including imagery, metaphor, emotion regulation, movement, posture, and sensory experience.

10. Self-processes in CBT foster metacognitive awareness as well as the accessing and building of wise and compassionate self-states for navigating the challenges posed by cancer.

11. A focus on strength, resilience, and meaning adds dignity and direction to clinical work with cancer patients.

12. A more contextual account of human functioning allows for a richer understanding of human change processes as well as for understanding those processes that maintain human suffering.

Three
Opening Moves and Session Structure in CBT for Cancer Patients

The challenges of creating and maintaining a psychotherapeutic treatment relationship with cancer patients can be nuanced and complex. Depending upon the phase of treatment and the nature of the disease, a high level of distress can be quite normal and is not necessarily an indication that the patient wants to discuss his or her emotional experience. Patient distress occurring early in the diagnosis and treatment phase may be best addressed by rapid engagement in curative or life prolonging medical treatments (Baker et al., 2013). In turn, the therapeutic engagement strategies employed by providers may differ according to their role and discipline. Forsey et al. (2013) found that physicians prefer a more instrumental and emotionally non-overt way of communicating to parents of children with leukemia. In contrast, nurses, who are not as directly involved in providing curative efforts, tended to prefer a more emotionally engaged style of communication. Patients may be quite satisfied with the more direct and instrumental forms of communication from their doctors, yet be more receptive to emotional support from others on the care team. Finally, there is evidence that the patient's attachment style, especially involving views of self, influences how well supported he or she feels in relation to his or her medical providers (Harding et al., 2015). Behavioral health clinicians working with cancer patients need to be aware of the importance of these issues, to more carefully titrate emotionally evocative material, as indicated by patient need and preference, and by phase of medical treatment. CBT and DBT have developed models that are well suited to addressing the relational needs of cancer patients, both in terms of phase of cancer treatment, and in terms of dealing with patients who may be predisposed to self-invalidation and trust concerns, and who may find emotional expression to be threatening.

In his original treatment manual for depression, Aaron Beck wrote that before becoming a good Cognitive Therapist, one had to first be a good psychotherapist (A. Beck & Rush, 1979). Somehow, as the model was disseminated, the meaning of that lesson may have been lost. In my work with clinicians around the United States, and in the way that CBT is sometimes characterized by adherents of other therapies, CBT is often depicted in a way that I do not recognize. It is often depicted as driven by a focus on techniques, rather than a focus on the person; by a simplistic belief that CBT involves forcing people to think differently; and by a rigidly manualized treatment protocol.

Yes, CBT is focused on helping free people from limited, inflexible, and at times inaccurate ways of viewing self and world. However, as Safran and Segal (1990) wrote,

> At the first sign that the patient does not appear to be open to an alternative construction of reality, the therapist should stop in the midst of the intervention and begin to explore precisely what is going on for the patient at that moment.
>
> (p. 89)

If the patient has pulled away, due to feeling misunderstood or invalidated by the therapist, the therapy repairs the relationship before anything else. CBT does not force change on people. In fact, when done by skilled practitioners, CBT offers a compassionate, safe, and respectful relationship, steeped in many of the humanistic principles outlined long ago by Carl Rogers (Rogers, 1951; 1980).

Having had the chance to watch therapeutic masters in many different forms of therapy, in all cases, one thing shone: the therapist was engaged, fully present, and caring. Something sparkled. There was warmth, appropriate humor, and encouragement to find a path out of suffering, even in the most difficult of circumstances. And in every encounter, if the observer has a sufficient understanding of the therapy model being employed, the particulars of the treatment model are readily apparent, and clearly serve to organize the session through the disciplined use of the therapist's self. Christine Padesky has written about her early experiences training with Beck. She writes that the first time she saw Beck conduct an interview, she did not see the techniques or session structure clearly, leading her to believe that perhaps Beck was himself not an effective practitioner of his own model. It was only as she gained experience with the model that she came to see how the model showed up in a very disciplined way when he worked, in what otherwise appeared to be just a warm and friendly conversation between two people (Salkovskis, 1996b).

Indeed, the patient's perception of the treatment relationship is positively related to treatment outcome, more so than the specific model of therapy employed (Norcross & Lambert, 2013). This recognition of the importance of relationship factors, and other non-specific factors, may lead some to believe that the specific treatment model is not important. However, Wampold and Impel, who have been critical of some aspects of the evidence-based therapy movement, wrote,

Training that focuses on treatments and ignores relationship skills, ignores the research evidence about what makes therapy effective. But it is also detrimental for trainees to learn relationship skills to the exclusion of learning particular approaches to psychotherapy. *The optimal training programs will combine training in treatments and relationships skills—this is a scientific approach to training* [emphasis added].

(Wampold & Imel, 2015, p. 276)

Novice and intermediate therapists often model themselves on their mentors or on the masters they observe in the therapies they are learning. At the expert level, however, the model and its techniques are all one's own, blending seamlessly with the person of the therapist. There appears to be nothing forced and no artifice. Two expert practitioners of the same model may appear very different in the way they work, but if you look carefully, the model still organizes their efforts. I've seen seasoned clinicians moved to tears watching a video of Aaron "Tim" Beck creating hope and connection in an interview with a young man struggling with psychosis. If you watch other masters of CBT, you will see very different personalities, yet all clearly and discernibly using the Cognitive Therapy model. And the same is true of seasoned ACT or DBT practitioners. At heart, what is on display, besides the theory and techniques of the model, is what Linehan has described as Level 6 validation, *Radical Genuineness* (Linehan, 1997). A student of Martin Buber said about him: "When he sat with you, he gave you his full attention. Only you existed. This ability to listen and to give you the feeling that he was waiting for you, as you are, influenced people" (Friedman, 1991, p. 334). Working with cancer patients provides the therapist not only the chance to be helpful but also the opportunity for personal and professional growth, to become more radically genuine, accepting, and compassionate toward ourselves and others. This can set the stage for our patients to more safely experience and express the pain they are in and to find a path.

Guided Discovery and Socratic Questioning

In the model presented here, disciplined listening and inquiry is at the heart of creating a treatment relationship as well as in generating a case formulation for treatment of cancer patients. Two sets of methods will be highlighted for this: Guided Discovery and Socratic Questioning (GD/SQ), from Beck's CBT, and Validation strategies, from DBT. They can dovetail seamlessly.

Guided Discovery is a collaborative process that

can be regarded as an overarching strategy that underpins many uses of skills in CBT. It refers to the way CBT therapists seek to facilitate clients' movement from less functional/flexible patterns of thinking, feeling and doing, toward more functional/flexible ones.

(Wills, 2015, p. 64)

The use of Socratic Questions is intended to help our patients access experience and to verbalize it, as well as examine it, for purposes of finding what works and what does not work toward achieving purposes and goals in specific problem situations. It does not force change on people, by trying to change minds (Padesky, 1993), or by presuming to know better than the patient what is true or what will work for the patient. Mark Reinecke has described the softer style of Guided Discovery and Socratic Questioning thusly:

> I don't presume that I have any access to truth. All I presume is that the way that the client is thinking about things isn't quite working for them. So it's a very gentle enquiry: I am just wondering if there is another way of thinking about it. But the essence of it then is the targeting of a specific maladaptive core belief and a gentle encouragement to sort of—I put my hand up like this—to turn the prism in the light and see if there's another angle from which it can be understood.
>
> (Kazantzis et al., 2014, p. 10)

Guided Discovery and Socratic Questioning invites exploration and collaboration. It invites a clear look at roadblocks and resources for dealing with the challenges that brought the patient to us for help. And the path to this understanding involves accessing and following emotionally evocative cognition, or hot cognition. A wise trout guide once explained to me that most casts into a stream are wasted effort. Trout congregate in richly oxygenated water, or in deeper pools. To find the trout, he said, "follow the bubbles in the stream." The bubbles in the stream of therapy are linked to emotion.

The sequence tends to involve the following:

1. Accessing information about current problems and maintaining factors, of which the patient may be unaware;
2. Reflecting back what we have heard, in order to insure our accurate understanding;
3. Summarizing the material we have gathered in session;
4. Synthesizing and helping generate new alternatives for thinking, experiencing, and acting (Wills, 2015).

DBT validation strategies dovetail with Guided Discovery and Socratic Questioning techniques to achieve the above sequence in therapy sessions. DBT's validation strategies were developed to address the challenges of working with patients with borderline personality disorder (Linehan, 1993a; 1997). Validation strategies are used here because they support the process of normalizing patient distress in the context of current circumstances and, at times, the patient's life history. To review the levels of validation:

Level 1 Validation involves listening with full attention to the patient;
Level 2 involves an acknowledgment that one has heard the patient, through one's words, gestures, and posture;

Level 3 occurs when the therapist gives voice to the thoughts, emotions, or
   behavior patterns which the patient has not yet verbalized;

Level 4 validates current emotions, thoughts, and behavior in terms of their
   historical causes;

Level 5 validates thoughts, urges, emotions, and behaviors as valid in the
   current context;

Level 6 Radical Genuineness validates and affirms the person, his or her
   worth as a human being, without regard to the emotions, thought, or
   behavior patterns that the person brings to therapy.

DBT validation principles help normalize and make sense of one's experience,
while setting the stage for acceptance and change. In addition, the therapist can help
maintain a balance between emotion exposure and downregulating emotion, as
appropriate. Validation, delivered in a systematic and targeted manner, can decrease
emotional and psychophysiological arousal. A therapist who uses DBT validation
strategies and Guided Discovery in a disciplined, targeted manner, may help downregulate painful emotions and reduce emotional and psychophysiological reactivity, in session. This, in turn, promotes the therapy relationship and aids in cueing
more adaptive emotions and responses to distress. Emotion regulation is related to
effective problem solving, including health outcomes (Gottman & Levenson, 1992),
and is facilitated by interpersonal validation. Laboratory studies of validating and
invalidating responses in experimental conditions demonstrate the effects on emotional reactivity. Invalidating conditions are related to heightened and sustained
reactivity involving negative affect and increased heart rate and skin conductance in
non-clinical samples (Shenk & Fruzzetti, 2011). Highly emotionally aroused cancer
patients, particularly when encountering invalidating responses from intimate others or the medical team, may experience an exacerbation of emotional reactivity, on
top of the fear arousal occasioned by the diagnosis of cancer itself.

   Kelly Koerner (2012) wrote, "When you validate, accurately and with precision,
you not only reduce arousal but also trigger competing responses" (p. 116). In fact,
validation *is* a change strategy, as compelling as the more technological elements
that are part of the cognitive and behavior therapies. Koerner wrote:

> It is tempting to view change strategies . . . as the main engine of therapy,
> the most important part of the help you offer, as if behavior therapy were a
> crowbar that needs a counterweight of validation to pry the patient toward
> change. But these views are wrong-headed and simplistic. They miss the pow-
> erful change that validation, *in itself*, produces.
>
> (Koerner, 2012, p. 111)

Opening Moves Example

The following is an example of the opening moves, in the first session with a cancer patient. Notice that there is no outward effort to change the patient's thinking,

behavior patterns, or interpersonal functioning. Yet notice, too, what change may be effected by using GD/SQ and validation, not as a trick, but from a place of genuineness. The disciplined use of GD/SQ and validation strategies conveys to the patient that we are listening, we understand, and that their responses make sense, given both their history and their current circumstances. As we will see in subsequent chapters, however, validation of the person does not necessarily mean validation of the strategies they are employing in dealing with cancer.

The patient is a 35-year-old woman, Caitlin, newly diagnosed with breast cancer, referred by her medical oncologist, and presenting for help with what she calls overwhelming anxiety, and a fear that her husband will leave her after her mastectomy, which is scheduled for the following week.

THERAPIST: So it sounds like you're worried about the surgery, and then about how your husband will handle this?

CAITLIN: I can't believe this is all happening! (Takes tissues out of her purse)

THERAPIST: Caitlin, I can see how difficult this is for you. It's so sudden, to be adjusting to all of this. If you want, we'll all help you get through this, all of our team here. (Validation levels 1 & 2, and offer of emotional and practical support)

CAITLIN: This is so scary. It's all happened so fast. I can't even get my mind around all of this. Sometimes I just can't even think straight.

THERAPIST: Anybody would be scared when they face surgery. I'm guessing that right now, it's not only the surgery; it's all kinds of things that are worrying you, like you are experiencing so many worries that your mind and emotions are just spinning (Levels 3 & 5 validation)

CAITLIN: Spinning is right. That's exactly what I feel like, like I'm spinning so fast I'm dizzy all the time.

THERAPIST: Yeah. Worry will do that to us, especially when we face a big health threat. If we could take some time to sort out all the worries that are passing through your mind, maybe one at a time, I'm thinking we could find a way to deal with them. What do you say we see what we can do? (Normalizing worry in context, level 5 validation, offer of problem-solving focus)

CAITLIN: (Nods yes) I think that would be a good idea.

THERAPIST: OK. Can I make a guess or two here? (Asks permission for level 3 validation)

CAITLIN: (Nods yes)

THERAPIST: I'm thinking it's not just the surgery you're worrying about. You said your family has a history of cancer. And you're worried about how your husband will handle this? (Level 3 validation)

CAITLIN: Yeah. Those are two big worries.

THERAPIST: Which one would you like to talk about first? Which one seems more important right now? (Moves to create problem list and set agenda collaboratively with patient)

CAITLIN: (Making eye contact) My mom died of breast cancer. My aunt died of it. What if, after everything, I don't make it? That's my biggest fear.

THERAPIST: (Briefly silent) You mean that you'll go through all the surgery, and whatever follow-up chemo or radiation you need, and still won't make it through this?

CAITLIN: (Nods) Yeah. That I'll have to deal with getting my breasts cut off, going through chemo, losing my hair, and dying. Like my mom did.

THERAPIST: Given what your mom went through, I can see why that fear might be in your mind right now. (Level 4 validation) Does anyone else know this is your big fear? (Therapist elects to target aloneness and social support, rather than either further validate fears in the context of the patient's history of mother's death or move to assess for presence of cognitive biases, which seemed premature.)

CAITLIN: No. I can't talk about that with anyone. When I bring it up with my husband, he switches the subject fast. So does my dad, and so do my brothers and sisters. Nobody wants to face the possibility that I could die. Even my oncologist seems freaked out. He just says not to think about dying, that he'll tell me if and when I have anything to worry about.

THERAPIST: I am sitting here imagining what that's like for you, to not feel that others have heard your fears about this. That you can't talk with anyone. I'm thinking that must feel lonely and scary. But I'm not sure what's there for *you*. (Levels 6 & 3 validation, and checking in with patient to confirm or modify)

CAITLIN: Yeah. Alone. And scared. I feel alone. I mean, I know they're all scared, too, especially my husband; but I just feel like I'm comforting *them*, protecting them, and I want someone to be able to hear *me*. Plus, there's something else. I'm really worried that when I get the mastectomy, my husband won't want to look at me. I won't have any breasts. Even if they do reconstruction, it won't be the same, and sometimes the reconstruction fails. My husband keeps saying he'll think I'm beautiful no matter what. But he hasn't seen what I've seen when my mom had a double mastectomy. He had an affair 2 years ago, and I can see him straying again after this.

THERAPIST: You know, it's beginning to make a lot of sense to me that you're feeling so stressed and vulnerable. I mean, let's look at the whole picture here. You're dealing with cancer. And you saw your mom die of this disease. You have major surgery that's coming up next week, which will leave you without your breasts, until the reconstruction is done, and you aren't sure the reconstruction will be successful. Given your fear of doctors, and maybe the fear that in the end, they don't help, it makes sense that you'd be so upset, doesn't it? You're spending time reassuring everyone around you and feel as though there's nobody there who understands *you*. And finally, after all this, you're worried that your husband will have another affair because he won't be attracted to you anymore. Do I have the whole picture here? Or is there something else I'm not understanding yet? (Capsule summary of what has transpired thus far in session, with levels 4 & 5 validation, followed by invitation for patient to confirm or modify)

CAITLIN: No. That's the whole picture. I think you've got it. Well maybe there's the issue with my oncologist, too. Even the doctor seems freaked out. Like he doesn't even want me to bring up my concerns about dying yet.

THERAPIST: OK, I think I'm getting a sense of what you've been feeling so overwhelmed by. The oncologist is part of what's troubling you, too. So if we add that to the mix, it's making some sense here that you're feeling pretty scared and overwhelmed. (Simplified restatement of capsule summary, after patient confirmation; Level 5 validation)

CAITLIN: Yeah. When you put it that way, it makes sense. I hadn't put all that into words before. Now that we've talked, I'm still really scared, but at least I feel like we've sort of mapped out the terrain a little bit. And I do feel better just talking about it with you. (Breathes deeply, sits back in chair)

THERAPIST: I also think that there's a path through this terrain. You've gone through a lot of challenges, and it sounds like you have always found a way to deal with what life has thrown at you. I'm not sure yet exactly what the path through this will look like, but if you want, we can find it together. Maybe I can help you find the compass inside you, and if you want, we'll find the path through this terrain together. (Patient's physical release of tension, noted in posture and breath, cues therapist to set a provisional course for therapy. Drawing on the patient's metaphor of having mapped out the terrain, the therapist utilizes the metaphor to invite the patient to consider that CBT and the relationship provides a compass and a path out, though the therapist does not have to know or say what that path might be at this point. He or she cannot know. That will emerge from the collaboration between therapist and patient.)

CAITLIN: (Smiles) I'd like that.

Session Summary

The first part of this session was devoted to engagement and GD/SQ and validation strategies. Change took the form in this session of a dampening in the patient's emotional reactivity, following the chance to be understood and to make sense of her experience. No effort was made to challenge or directly change the patient's thinking or her coping strategies. The therapist followed the trail of emotion, helping the patient implicitly ride her fear, rather than be ridden by it. The therapist generated hypotheses that can be used later for therapeutic interventions. For example, we might ask the patient to rate her conviction that she, like her mother, will die. She could engage in a behavioral experiment, testing her beliefs, or testing a new strategy for dealing with her oncologist, in order to get a sense of what the facts are regarding her prognosis. At the same time, it will be important for the therapist and the team to provide assurances of non-abandonment, no matter what the course of her disease (Levin & Applebaum, 2012). We also do not know how accurately or functionally she might be reading her relationship with her husband, in terms of his response to her upcoming mastectomy and the tenuousness of their relationship. The therapist will use GD/SQ to explore this in greater detail later, both to refine hypotheses about problems and maintaining factors and to select techniques. Last, the stage was set create a problem list and a therapy agenda.

Joining

With time at a premium, with heavy caseloads, and with a highly technology focused delivery system, the human dimension of care can be impaired (Ofri, 2005; Gawande, 2015). Even in visits with behavioral health professions, rating scales, forms requesting information about presenting problems, and alcohol, drug, and developmental histories may precede the first visit. Taking the time to get to know the patient and any accompanying family members is often vital, and it sets the stage for effective therapeutic work.

Joining strategies can help. "Joining" is a term that originated in the work of Salvador Minuchin's Structural Family Therapy (Minuchin, 1974; Minuchin et al., 1978; Minuchin & Fishman, 1981; Lindblad-Goldberg et al., 1989). Taking even 5 minutes to ask about a person's life can not only be highly validating, but also provide a safe haven in the midst of cancer therapy, spark trust in the therapist, motivate the patient, generate relevant hypotheses and metaphors, and ease the path toward setting a therapy agenda. Effective CBTers use a form of joining, as anyone who has watched Beck work knows. However, making it a deliberate, disciplined strategy, as with validation strategies and GS/SQ, expands the customary CBT framework to good effect. Many patients who present for psychological help in cancer centers may have had no prior experience with a psychologist, psychiatrist, or clinical social worker. It can be a frightening experience in and of itself and is often fraught with expectations that they will be scrutinized, objectified, diagnosed, and deemed in need of serious re-tooling as a person. Joining allows the therapist to ease the person into the encounter, without sacrificing time spent in generating clinically relevant information about strengths, values, hopes, and daily life.

John Gregory, 65, and his wife, Adrianne, 58, arrive for a first visit together. John is a newly retired machinist at a farm implement manufacturing company in a small town in southern Iowa. Adrianne still works as a secretary at a local elementary school. John presents with a recurrence of skin cancer, affecting his left ear and now the scalp. He has had surgery, which involved removal of part of his ear, plastic surgery to reconstruct the ear, and then radiation therapy of his head. Now, the cancer has developed on the scalp behind his other ear. Prior to beginning a new course of radiation therapy, he is also seeing oral surgery, to assess whether teeth need to be removed in the radiation field, prior to starting radiation therapy. His wife is concerned that John is becoming depressed and withdrawn. Before asking about depression and anxiety problems, the therapist makes an effort to join with John and Adrianne.

THERAPIST:	You had a long drive here today, didn't you?
JOHN:	Yep. We were up at 5 a.m. and on the road by a quarter to 6.
THERAPIST:	You drove in from where?
JOHN:	Winterset (John Wayne's birthplace)
THERAPIST:	Winterset! John Wayne country, right?
JOHN:	(Smiling) It sure is. Have you been to the museum there?
THERAPIST:	Not yet.
JOHN:	Well, you ought to come down there. It's really something. (Adrianne speaks next)
ADRIANNE:	That's not all we have there. We have the Bridges of Madison County, like in the movie.
THERAPIST:	You're from there, too?
ADRIANNE:	No, I come from another little town. I moved to Winterset to be with John. This is a second marriage for each one of us. And he dragged me into Winterset. But I'm happy there now.

(What follows is a discussion of the bridges of Madison County, Iowa, the natural beauty of the rolling hills, especially in the fall, when the trees are yellow, gold, and red. The couple enjoys fall outings together and talk about their favorite secluded and beautiful places, where they sometimes picnic or take walks together. John and Adrianne invite the therapist to visit them the next time she passes through the area.)

In the 5 minutes of such a conversation, not only can patients be put at ease, but also patients can see the therapist as a person such as them, one who is genuinely curious about their lives and is perhaps interested in some of the same things that interest the patients. In addition, a wealth of data can be generated about the person's life history, strengths and resources, phase of life concerns, and key relationships. While listening to patient narratives, potential hot cognitions can be spotted and potential cognitive biases, or behavior patterns that may be implicated in problem maintenance, can emerge. All of this information can be drawn from in forming hypotheses about maintaining factors, problem lists, case conceptualizations, and interventions later.

Fostering a Change Agenda

Creating a validating, warm, and empathic treatment environment is itself healing. Emotional expression, in the context of a validating relationship, is potentially calming and comforting in itself. Sometimes that is sufficient for a therapy encounter. But, in most cases, that is only part of the agenda in CBT. Helping the patient effect changes, via acceptance or change strategies, is a core part of the model. And in line with Linehan's description of Radical Genuineness, the therapist must find ways to invite the patient into an effort to think, do, and experience life either in new ways or by re-invoking older, functional adaptive patterns that may have been swamped by distress. DBT walks a dialectical line between two poles. On the one hand, DBT validates the logic of the patient's patterns of functioning, in light of the person's history, their current circumstances, and their emotional, cognitive, and behavioral repertoires. On the other hand, DBT specifically, and effective therapy more generally, does not validate coping strategies that are damaging. James Gustafson, director of the brief therapy clinic at the University of Wisconsin, said "the doctor's job is to make the unpleasant implications clear" (Gustafson, 1992, p. 17). Our job is to make those implications clear in ways that are inviting and that convey our belief that the patient has the resources and wisdom to find a path through their pain.

We are always maintaining a balance between acceptance and change, between validating and accepting the patient as they are, and guiding them toward change. CBT has long recognized that we can err on the side of pushing for change before the patient is ready for change, and that in so doing, we can spark a rupture in the treatment relationship. Safran and Segal (1990) provided a guide to noticing treatment ruptures and rectifying them. As a general rule, I advocate understanding the patient first, then fostering change later. But this balancing act is fraught with challenges, and as therapists we sometimes do not get it right. Noticing patient reactions when a rupture occurs, checking in with the patient, and rectifying the rupture is often all that is necessary to get the therapy back on track. Like the analyst Winnicott (1987) said, we needn't be perfect, just "good enough." Part of being good enough is tuning in to the relationship and working collaboratively with the patient to insure that we remain in lockstep about the therapy.

Creating a Session Structure

At heart, effective therapy is *about* something. Whether it is the initial provision of emotional support, making sense out of painful experiences, defining problems in a way that allows for acceptance and change, CBT is focused and provides a flexible structure for organizing each session. Session structure provides a consistent mechanism for the patient to be understood, to learn new, emotionally evocative information about themselves, and to more effectively address the problems for which they are seeking help. Structure is an ally, not a pair of handcuffs, and the skilled therapist learns with practice how to maintain a collaborative, conversational tone, while broadly adhering to the elements of a session's structure. This begins by making therapy about something that is of deep importance to the patient. While we work to enhance a sense of well-being and reduce suffering, perhaps a more powerful way of working is to set a course for therapy that is based on more enduring and meaningful life values, even in the face of distress (Hayes et al., 2001; Dahl et al., 2009; Wilson & DuFrene, 2009).

The following are guidelines for how a session is structured. These serve as standard elements in the structure of Beck's model of CBT (J. Beck, 2011a; Westbrook et al., 2012; Wills & Sanders, 2013; Wills, 2015).

1. Check-in and update
2. Bridge from prior session

3. Homework review
4. Setting an agenda
5. Session work
6. Taking new learning into daily life: setting homework
7. Capsule summaries and take-away points from session.

Check-in and update: It is useful in follow-up sessions to check in regarding what has transpired between sessions. For cancer patients, this can include a brief discussion about what new findings have emerged, how treatment has proceeded, what side effects are emerging from treatment, and what new psychological and/or interpersonal challenges have occurred. In working with depressed patients, it is also customary to get a mood rating, which can involve something as simple as a number, from 1 to 10, reflecting mood during the past week and/or in session today. The check-in can also include elements of joining, including information about how the patient's life is unfolding in non-problem areas. This might include discussion of meaningful and/or pleasurable activities or events that have occurred since the last session. This might include a visit from an adult child and grandchildren, to a fishing trip with an old friend, or a romantic night with one's partner. Time can be spent unfolding these experiences in a conversational manner. In addition, the therapist is vigilant for indications of fresh problems and challenges as well as a sense of whether a homework assignment from the last session was achieved.

Bridge from prior session: As part of the check-in, the therapist inquires about reactions to the last session, including lingering issues or concerns from the last meeting, including negative reactions that might have occurred. One can also inquire about what the patient was thinking about today's session on the way to the office. This can sometimes reveal reactions from the past session, reactions to the therapist, avoidance issues, or eagerness to discuss fresh issues in session.

Homework review: If there were a better word than "homework," I would use it. The key idea is to create an assignment, with the patient's full collaboration and willingness, which allows for and of the following: mindful observing and noticing, information gathering, testing of new ways of experiencing target situations, new ways of thinking about and reacting to problem situations, graduated exposure to fear situations, practicing new behavior patterns and problem-solving strategies, and building alternatives to avoidance, escape, or withdrawal. The list of specific homework tasks is potentially endless and involves both the collaboration and creativity of the therapist and patient. At heart, homework involves the patient either observing, gathering data, or doing more or less of a specific behavior in a target situation. Once a homework assignment has been developed, it must be followed up on in the next session. Failing to check on a homework assignment in the next session damages the relationship and derails the therapy.

Setting an agenda: Given the frequently short duration of therapy with cancer patients, time efficiency is vital. We begin formulating a list of problems the patient faces, in terms that are specific and that can become the focus for therapeutic interventions. Listening during the check-in for new problems that have arisen, as well as which of the existing problems are most salient, sets the stage for creating a session agenda. It is wise to preserve an overall agenda that guides the entire therapy, while also being sensitive to the need to alter the course of therapy on the basis of patient need. Focusing on the collaborative nature of the treatment relationship prevents too rigid an approach to structuring the therapy, including agenda setting. It is wise to select one item, two at most, to address in the session, leaving time to do the work of the session and to find a fresh assignment that allows the patient to take today's learning into daily life.

Session work: The bulk of the session involves addressing the specific agenda item and its relevance to the problem at hand. We may focus on the maintaining factors preventing effective adaptation to the problem at hand as well as working to modify those maintaining factors. The full spectrum of techniques available in the CBT family of therapies and beyond is available, like a broad range of colors on a painter's palette. Freud once famously said that therapy was akin to chess, in that the opening moves and end games are well documented and can be easily learned, "while the middle game can only be acquired by actual practice and contact with the great masters" (Freud, 1958, p. 123). Cognitive behavior therapy takes a middle road in this: by developing an effective case conceptualization, the therapist is able to pinpoint maintaining factors that impede effective coping, and by targeting the core processes implicated in problem maintenance, appropriate techniques can be selected to help the patient.

Taking new learning into daily life: setting homework: Capsule summaries are embedded in the session frequently, as we have seen, in order to insure that the patient is being understood, and to help set the stage for framing a change agenda. The therapist concludes each session by asking for feedback about what was accomplished, if the therapy has met the patient's objectives, and if there were any moments or experiences in session that troubled the patient. This, in addition to tuning in to non-verbal behavior suggestive of negative reactions to therapist interventions, allows for breaches in the therapy relationship to be addressed in a way that hopefully limits premature termination (Newman, 2013).

Capsule summaries and take-away points from session: One of the common challenges in CBT is knowing how and when to begin shifting the focus of a session from doing the work that forms the bulk of the session to designing an assignment that takes the work of the session into the patient's daily life. Therapists who master this step begin thinking about this well before the session ends so that ample time can be allotted for this step to unfold successfully. I advise thinking in terms of the following:

1. Set up homework as a no-lose process; information gained is valuable no matter what.
2. What are the processes maintaining the problems that are most susceptible to change?
3. How big a step does the patient appear able or willing to take?
4. Are we setting our sights on observing, collecting data, or practicing new ways of coping in vivo in our assignment?
5. What might get in the way of taking that step this week?

6. What is the patient's buy-in and ownership of the assignment?
7. Get patient summary of the assignment.
8. What is the likelihood of completion?
9. Re-design if necessary, to insure a high probability of completion.

Clinicians new to the model often struggle with how to maintain the pace necessary to adhere to a session structure. It is possible for the treatment relationship to suffer as clinicians new to the model struggle to be adherent. But with disciplined effort, including supervision, session structure becomes an ally and can be flexibly applied. Frank Wills wrote:

> In his various demonstrations of therapy, live or in recorded sessions, Beck shows that it is possible to wear the structure lightly. He also implies that the prime structure is in the internal template of where therapy is moving, rather than in a series of rigid behavioural steps.
>
> (Wills, 2009 p. 111)

At the expert level, session structure is readily discernible to the observer, but it tends to be gentler and it fits comfortably with the style and personality of the therapist. It is akin to the structure of a jazz performance, in which improvisation occurs around the chord, melodic, and rhythmic structure of the overall composition. Once the clinician becomes adept at incorporating structure into his or her repertoire, flexibility, based on patient need, is easily achieved. To again quote Frank Wills, "while in general a structured approach offers clients the best deal, it is sometimes important for the therapist to respond strongly to the client's individual needs, which may be for structure but also for toning down structure" (Wills, 2009, p. 111). A patient who arrives to the session just after learning that cancer has spread, despite chemotherapy, needs compassion and support first, not a review of last session's homework. Yet even in such situations, it becomes possible to help the patient re-enter the structure of a session, to address steps to be taken to manage the sad news just received. Another key element in the session structure is the way that structure allows the patient to learn about the CBT model and about expectations for how the therapy might unfold, including the responsibilities of both the patient and the therapist for setting a course of treatment. Research regarding the therapy's effectiveness is employed to inform the patient about the model's evidence base as well as to encourage patient adherence in order to secure the best possible outcome.

Case Example

Russ Szymanski is a 53-year-old married father of two adult sons, one of whom works with him in his family auto parts business. The company has grown substantially and now has 38 employees, located in three cities. Russ was recently diagnosed with a head and neck cancer, for which surgery took place, followed by radiation therapy, which is now in progress. He is fatigued and in pain much of the time. Yet despite the effects of cancer, he insists on maintaining his customary work pace, even with daily radiation therapy. He works more than 70 hours a week, and travels between stores, which requires additional driving time, since the company has stores in three cities in the state. His son, age 29, is ostensibly being groomed to eventually become CEO, although Russ has been loath to relinquish the control of daily operations. Russ grew up in a family in which his father was a violent alcoholic, who lost job after job, and died when Russ was 11, leaving Russ's mom to raise Russ and his two younger sisters. Russ developed a profound sense of personal responsibility for his mother and his younger sisters, and to this day he maintains financial responsibilities to them all. His youngest sister married an alcoholic, and they are in constant financial distress, frequently turning to Russ to lend them money that they never repay. He is contributing to the college education of his other sister's oldest daughter, and he supports his mother, who is elderly, ill, and unable to drive. His sense of personal responsibility extends into his marriage, his role as a father, and his sense of responsibility for his employees and their families.

His loyalty to others and his sense of personal responsibility are strengths. However, the implicit rules and assumptions governing his life are among the maintaining factors in his current dilemma. He is getting increasingly exhausted, sleep deprived, and unable to focus effectively on the many challenges he is facing. He believes that he must nonetheless maintain the work pace he maintained at age 30, and the financial responsibilities he maintains for others. They include such rules and assumptions as, "If I don't keep going, everyone who depends on me will suffer"; "I need to be Superman; everyone has come to see me that way, and I can't let them down"; "Without me, the company will fail, and everyone who depends on me will be out of jobs"; "If I don't look in on my mom every day, she'll be alone"; "My wife depends on me for emotional support; I'll be weak if I lean on her right now."

Acting on the previous rules and assumptions has contributed to exhaustion, loneliness, a sense of isolation, business difficulties, and an inability or unwillingness to ask for support and practical assistance in any major endeavor of his life. Mr. Szymanski faced weeks of continued radiation therapy as well as the possibility of more surgery. The session uncovered Mr. Syzmanski's strongly held conviction that he must be "Superman" and that relinquishing any area of perceived personal responsibility would be viewed by him as a sign of personal weakness and failure. There was one area, however, in which he was willing to consider asking for help: his mother. He recognized that his sister had more time and could be more involved in helping their mother with daily needs. He also, more abstractly, recognized that it would be wise to ask his son to assume slightly greater responsibility for the company, even on a temporary basis. The therapist explored a homework assignment that might address each:

THERAPIST: So if you were to take a step, one that is maybe a test, to see if your sister could step up to this challenge, what might it be?

RUSS: I don't know. I go over to mom's probably five days a week, even if it's for a few minutes. Lisa (Russ's wife) goes over there, too. My sister lives in town, but she kind of relies on Lisa and me to take care of mom's grocery shopping and stuff like that.

THERAPIST: And what's your sister's name?

RUSS: Carol.

THERAPIST: OK, so Carol helps a little bit, but not too much. Does she recognize how much mom needs right now, and what you're going through?

RUSS: I think so. Finally. But she's always looked to me to make things right, and to take care of everyone, including her. I send money to her every month, especially when her husband is out of work, like he is now.

THERAPIST: He's the drinking man?

RUSS: (Nods head) He's the one, I'm afraid.

THERAPIST: OK, so maybe this could be a chance for Carol to do a little more for her mom, and especially now for her big brother. Do you think her big brother needs and could handle having Carol step up? (Therapist encourages patient to view self from a distance here, and reflect on his needs more dispassionately) And maybe just as important, do you think Carol would have a stronger, maybe better sense of herself if she could contribute to her mom and big brother; like it'd be good for her and everyone if she stepped in to help here?

RUSS: (Momentarily silent) I never looked at it like that.

THERAPIST: Spoken like that Superman inside you. (Therapist draws on patient's prior metaphor for self as Superman) Only now, I'm thinking that maybe there's some kryptonite that's weakening you a bit. And so maybe it's not only you who need some support; it's Carol who needs to know she can help out her mom and brother here.

RUSS: That'd be a new twist on life. I never looked at it like that.

THERAPIST: Even Superman needs a helper sometimes. Lois Lane, Jimmy Olsen. Right?

RUSS: (Laughs) I guess it'd help everyone.

THERAPIST: So let's say you're not quite ready to let go of a lot of responsibility. You've already said that you're not sure Carol can live up to responsibilities. And I guess you've given good reasons for your skepticism. But if she and you need a chance to show she *can* take on some responsibilities here, what would be a step in that direction, one you could describe so I could see it in my mind's eye, along with you, so we could both see and hear it clearly?

RUSS: Hmm. Well, you know, I have an audit coming up in Cedar City, and it'd be helpful if Carol could take mom grocery shopping this week, instead of me or Lisa.

THERAPIST: OK. So let's walk through how you might approach her and get this outcome to happen, or at least make the effort, knowing there's something in it for you, your mom, and for your sister, too.

The therapist and the patient use problem-solving strategies and role plays to create a strategy that Russ agrees to implement later that day. Barriers to implementation seem few, and Russ conveys a sense of certainty that he will contact his sister. In addition, Russ understands that he does not control the outcome of this effort. It will be his sister's call. However, he does believe that Carol might willingly embrace the role of co-Superman or Superwoman and recognizes that cancer, as well as surgery and radiation therapy, has become his kryptonite, and that for now, at least, he needs to begin asking for support. If successful, this homework assignment might set the stage for not only appropriately asking for support from others but also for giving others in his life a chance to take responsibility and leadership roles as well. The change strategy was geared to the patient's need to reduce his workload, in the service of protecting himself and respecting the limits of his energy, given the demands of his intensive treatment. However, given his beliefs about self, and the rules by which he lives, he was loathe to step away from responsibilities, and the therapy focused on crafting the least change tolerable to him, as a way of edging him a step further toward respecting his current limitations, without lapsing into self-reproach. More regarding how to achieve these steps will follow in clinical chapters. For now, the central issue is the use of session structure, to insure that the therapist stay connected, gather relevant data, set an agenda, work the agenda, and create a clear step forward, to be taken between sessions.

Chapter Summary

This chapter focused on the role of the therapeutic relationship in working with cancer patients. Strategies to build an effective and genuinely engaged therapeutic relationship were presented, including Guided Discovery/Socratic Questions as well as DBT validation strategies. The two methods combine to allow for a disciplined set of strategies to build and maintain an effective therapy relationship. This sets the stage for helping patients openly face the emotional pain of having cancer, in a validating and compassionate environment, while setting the stage for here-and-now coping. Effective use of these strategies helps the therapist attune to breaches in the relationship and their rectification. Session structure, utilizing the structure of a Beckian CBT session, helps shape the therapy, in terms of its focus, the establishment of roles and expectations, the psychoeducation of the patient, the collaborative nature of the relationship, the pace and flow of the session, and a framework for setting treatment targets, and implementing change strategies. Structure worn lightly is advocated, though it is wise to work within the structure as a novice, until one is able to effectively incorporate session structure and techniques into one's personality as an expert.

Key Points

1. CBT rests on a foundation of respect for the patient, compassion, and faith in the person's capacity to find a path through life's challenges.
2. The disciplined self of the therapist can be honed through the use of Guided Discovery/Socratic Questions as well as DBT's validation strategies.
3. The therapist explores and validates the sometimes hidden logic of the patient's efforts to manage the problems either created by, or exacerbated by, cancer.
4. The therapist fosters an open expression and acceptance of the patient's suffering, while fostering here-and-now coping with the demands imposed by cancer and its treatment(s).
5. At the same time, the therapist is an advocate for the patient to use his or her strengths and resources to find new, more effective ways of meeting the challenges of cancer.
6. Key elements of the session structure include:
   a. Setting an agenda;
   b. Defining a key area for the session's focus;
   c. Addressing the factors that are maintaining the problem, or that are preventing more flexible and adaptive coping;
   d. Intervention design and implementation;
   e. Using the spectrum of evidence-based and theory-based interventions;
   f. Setting a homework assignment where feasible;
   g. Providing check-ins and capsule summaries, and eliciting feedback about the therapy.

Four
Creating Case Formulations for Work with Cancer Patients

Having described key elements of the therapeutic relationship, and how to structure a CBT session, we are ready to address the creation of a case formulation. A case formulation is like any good navigational tool. It lets us identify a destination and set a course. When we go astray, it helps us figure out where we are and how to get back on course to our destination. In cognitive behavior therapy, a formulation allows us to get beneath a general diagnosis, and to define key problems in living, in very specific terms. A good formulation allows us to generate clinically testable hypotheses about the cognitive, emotional, behavioral, and contextual factors that are maintaining the problems as well as hypotheses about the historical factors in the patient's life that create vulnerabilities in the here-and-now. Finally, we want to know what strengths and resources are available in the patient's historical repertoire and current environment, which can be brought to bear in dealing with life's challenges.

There is abundant literature on case formulations in CBT as well as numerous models from which to choose (Persons, 1989, 2008; Needleman, 1999; Kuyken et al., 2009; Kuyken et al., 2010; J. Beck, 2011a; Westbrook et al., 2012; Wills & Sanders, 2013; Bennett-Levy et al., 2015; Eells, 2015; Wills, 2015). If we broaden the focus to include other models from within the CBT family, both ACT and DBT have their own case formulation approaches (Linehan, 1993a; Hayes, Villatte, et al., 2011; Koerner, 2012). ACT formulations can be quite parsimonious (Hayes, Villatte et al., 2011; Strosahl et al., 2012; Strosahl et al., 2015), organized around a three-pillar approach, including "Open-Aware-Active," which assesses the degree to which the person maintains an open, accepting stance to experience; an awareness of the relevant internal and external processes implicated in problem maintenance; and an active stance toward committed, value-based, behavior change. In the case of Focused Acceptance and Commitment Therapy (FACT), the principles of Open-Aware-Active can be employed to begin shaping a case conceptualization in a single session and setting the stage for potentially rapid change (Strosahl et al., 2012).

While there is general agreement about the utility of case formulations in CBT, data regarding reliability and validity are equivocal. It appears that the more descriptive the formulation, such as creating a problem list, the higher the reliability. When the formulation addresses more speculative elements, reliability declines. This includes speculation about assumptions, core beliefs and schemas, and linkages to historical development. More experienced therapists may produce higher rates of reliability (Kuyken et al., 2009). Interested readers will find free access to a variety of case formulations and worksheets at www.psychologytools.com.

I will use a case formulation that draws mainly on the works of Persons (1989; 2008), Kuyken et al. (2009), and Wills (2015) in a way that allows for targeting and intervening in the entire range of cognitive, emotional, behavioral, and contextual processes identified in Chapter 2. Those factors appear in the following sections:

Transdiagnostic Factors

Cognitive
Cognitive Biases
Verbally encoded as well as implicitly encoded via metaphor, imagery, body
 sensation
Cognitive Processes
Worry
Rumination

Emotional
Emotion Dysregulation

Behavioral Processes
Problem-solving difficulties
Avoidance, escape, and safety-seeking behaviors

The aim here will be parsimony, simplicity, and ease of use. Formulations will be tailored for the fast-paced encounters that occur in cancer clinics, where acuity of suffering can be high, duration of therapy brief, and background information limited. Thorough case conceptualizations may require several sessions, and even then they always remain provisional and subject to revision on the basis of new data. Working in cancer clinics, however, often requires us to make a rapid formulation, with a clear problem list, and a focused intervention plan, beginning in the first session. Naturally, in such cases, we recognize the limits of our formulations' completeness and utility. With opportunities for longer episodes of therapy, or when therapy unfolds over a longer time frame, we can develop more detailed formulations. More elaborate formulations, involving more entrenched, complex maintaining processes, can be developed as necessity and time permit.

CBT case conceptualizations were initially developed for treatment of *DSM* disorders and are tailored to people caught in recurrent, dysfunctional patterns, or vicious cycles. Not all our patients are caught in long-standing vicious cycles. Certainly, for those patients with long-standing or pre-existing adaptive difficulties, a detailed formulation, including historical factors, is apt. Yet many cancer patients who present in the clinic may have strong adaptive histories, with substantial coping abilities. They are more likely to be experiencing adjustment difficulties, due to the sheer number of challenges imposed by the burdens of cancer. In some cases, patients may lack the flexibility to create new responses for current problems and find that their adaptive repertoire does not work in the current situation. But we can employ a formulation to rapidly map out the patient's response to cancer challenges nonetheless. In setting up lists of problems, we focus on not only broad diagnostic categories, such as depression and anxiety, but also a more fine-grained definition of problems. Problems consist of "a discrepancy between your current state (what is) and your desired state (what I want). This discrepancy is a problem because of the existence of various obstacles that block the path when trying to reach your goals" (Nezu et al., 2007, p. 4). This discrepancy is revealed through the use of validation strategies and Guided Discovery and Socratic Questioning (GD/SQ). For example, cancer fatigue is revealed to be a problem when the patient's fatigue is met with a belief such as "If I can't work full time, then I am a failure." It is not always intuitively obvious what makes something a problem for a person. For example, facing death has always struck me as a big problem. However, as I listened to my patients, I realized that dying in itself may not be the key problem for patients. Many patients have genuinely expressed a fearlessness about dying that has left an impact on me. Dying may become problematic when it is met by such meanings as "I'm afraid I'll die in pain"; "I don't want to be incapacitated and be a burden for a long time"; "If there is a God, I'm scared I'll be punished for not believing in him during my life"; "I'm afraid my family will not figure out how to repair the house if I die before the remodeling is done"; and "I don't want my wife, children and step-children to fight over my estate." Again, it is through the process of GD/SQ that we learn the private meanings, and the patterns in living, that create the discrepancy between what is and what one wants.

Figure 4.1 displays a quick but effective way of organizing clinical data when we know the patient is presenting in distress and when their own coping strategies are not working. If the patient is caught in a pattern of coping with cancer-related activating events that are contributing to distress, we can identify it as a vicious cycle. By the same token, we look for indications of patient strengths, which will help us work with them to create a virtuous cycle for the more effective navigation of their challenges (Butler et al., 2008). Safran and Segal (1990) cited multiple writers who have long recognized that vicious cycles are not just maintained

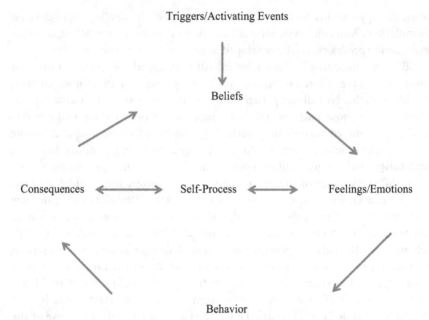

FIGURE 4.1 Vicious and Virtuous Cycles

Adapted from: F. Wills (2015). *Skills in Cognitive Behaviour Therapy (2nd Edition)*. London: Sage.

by cognition; they are interpersonal in nature, and as newer behavioral models have shown, they are maintained by their consequences, even when unhappiness is the paradoxical result. In fact, the vicious cycle model can be elaborated into an extended chain analysis, which maps in great detail problematic patterns, and their consequences, over a more extended time frame.

We begin with an Activating Event (AE), which may be linked to the reasons for the oncology team's referral to the behavioral health consultant. Since cancer is the common feature linking our patients to one another, we are attuned to cancer-related processes as activating events. These include disease site, stage of illness, effects of cancer, effects of treatment (such as pain and fatigue), or changes in body image and in key relationships. We then look into the beliefs, emotions, physical sensations, coping behaviors, and consequences that may be contributing to patient suffering. We then set out to explore the patient's thoughts, images, body sensations, emotions, behavior, and consequences of behavior. Each of those elements exists in a reciprocal relationship to one another. Influencing behavior can influence and change thoughts and can dampen or intensify emotion arousal. We can enter the cycle behaviorally or cognitively, to influence a fresh outcome of coping strategies. As we conduct this chain analysis, you will note that it is in the nature of a vicious cycle to get more of what you really don't want. A virtuous cycle tends to spark a sense of freedom, even in the midst of tough circumstances. The self-processes and behavioral repertoires implicated in vicious cycles lead to contraction; those in virtuous cycles are more flexible and expansive, engaging life as it is in a creative and purposeful manner.

As we generate clinical information for a formulation, we are going to be listening for, observing, and inquiring about the maintaining factors listed previously. One additional element in the formulation is the center: self-processes. These are not reducible to patient beliefs. Self-processes involve cognition and emotion, body sensations, images, memories, action urges, and behavioral and interpersonal patterns. Rationalist interventions may provide one route for accessing and altering these processes. Others include posture, movement, experiential exercises, guided imagery, behavioral experiments, and mindfulness practices.

Once we have a tentative idea about the pattern that is implicated in patient suffering, we can begin to create a case conceptualization and a treatment plan, drawing on a format designed by Persons (1989; 2008) and available at www.psychologytools.com. The following case formulation worksheet in Figure 4.2 provides a useful organizing tool for creating a rapid formulation and CBT treatment plan.

To illustrate these principles in action, let's return to a case from the Introduction, the case of Elvira, the 58-year-old depressed married mother of adult children, who presents with Stage IV colon cancer. She is facing the end of available treatments, and the eventual need for entry into hospice care. Despite pain and fatigue, Elvira still feels able to travel. She notes that her husband has been unsupportive, including of her wish to spend money on travel, even to visit children and grandchildren. Let's start by creating the beginning of a conceptualization for one key problem and one situation. We will be looking to find a potential vicious cycle of maintaining factors that is ensnaring Elvira in a pattern that is suggestive of possible depression. Then, we'll move on to create a formulation, using Figure 4.2.

Problem list	
1:	5:
2:	6:
3:	7:
4:	8:
Hypothesized mechanisms	
Relation of mechanisms to problems	
Triggers/precipitants for current problem	
Origins of mechanisms	
Strengths	
Treatment plan	

FIGURE 4.2 Case Formulation Worksheet

If we write a list of the problems Elvira faces, we would include an advanced, metastatic cancer; the end of active treatment and beginning of palliative care; a long-standing and unhappy marriage; her husband's seeming refusal or inability to collaborate in Elvira's wishes; financial problems; a wish to see her children and grandchildren while she is still capable of travel; health, husband, and financial barriers to travel; and depression, including withdrawal and isolation in the face of these challenges.

We next want to list the maintaining factors that are preventing Elvira from finding workable solutions to these problems. We discover that she has thoughts such as "I'm trapped," "I'll die before I can see my children and grandchildren," and "My husband doesn't care about me." She feels increasingly sad and depressed. As her mood drops, fatigue increases and pain worsens. Her behavioral response initially was to speak directly with her husband about her wishes. However, after trying once, and his refusal to pay for travel, Elvira withdrew silently into increased depression, pain and fatigue, and hopelessness and entrapment. By getting more detail, using the chain analysis (Koerner, 2012), we can see that her withdrawal was followed by her husband's becoming less irritable toward her. Elvira prefers peace, which she achieves by staying silent. But this peace comes at the cost of Elvira's deepening sense of being helpless, trapped, and fearful that she will die before she sees her children. Her withdrawal has become more generalized, however. She is now sitting alone in front of the TV, ruminating about how painful her life is for hours a day. Soon, she is also angry, resentful, and increasingly depressed. Figure 4.3 shows the vicious cycle of entrapment and hopelessness in which Elvira is becoming caught.

While generating the information obtained for Figure 4.3, we have made no immediate moves toward effecting change. Any probes we make are primarily to get a sense of how entrenched the person might be in their cognitive, emotional, and behavioral repertoire, especially in areas that are implicated in maintaining problems.

We are acquiring the clinical data we need to answer key questions and form clinically testable hypotheses:

1. What are the problems, and in what order might we focus on them?
2. What factors are maintaining the target problems and blocking Elvira's ability to solve the problems on her own?
3. What strengths does Elvira bring to the situation?
4. At what points in this vicious cycle might interventions lead to meaningful change?

We set up the problem list collaboratively, and we work with the patient to decide in what order we might address these problems. As we will see in Chapter 8, selecting target problems in very brief therapy requires a focus on what is possible, not necessarily on what is ideal. Then we design intervention strategies, trusting that a small, well-thought-out, focused step forward can create positive reverberating

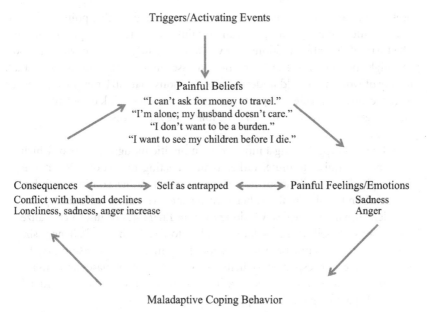

Triggers/Activating Events

Painful Beliefs
"I can't ask for money to travel."
"I'm alone; my husband doesn't care."
"I don't want to be a burden."
"I want to see my children before I die."

Consequences ⟷ Self as entrapped ⟷ Painful Feelings/Emotions
Conflict with husband declines   Sadness
Loneliness, sadness, anger increase   Anger

Maladaptive Coping Behavior

Withdrawal and isolation from contact with social supports
Avoids contact with husband
Rumination

FIGURE 4.3 Vicious Cycle: Elvira Mortensen

Adapted from: F. Wills (2015). *Skills in Cognitive Behaviour Therapy (2nd Edition)*. London: Sage.

effects in other areas of the person's life (Gustafson, 1992; 2005; Strosahl et al., 2012). James Gustafson said "many first steps are dead ends in a cul de sac, while a few first steps lead to continuous new beginnings" (personal communication, April 17, 2015).

Let's imagine the problem list we might set up with Elvira, to help her take a step into a continuous new beginning:

1. She is in an unhappy marriage.
2. The marital problems are exacerbating her current sense of isolation, entrapment, and hopelessness.
3. She is facing the end of the active treatment phase and a likely death from cancer at some point.
4. She wishes to see and spend time with her daughter and granddaughter, who live in another city, before she dies.
5. The couple has financial difficulties, worsened by her retirement from work, due to cancer.

We are gathering information that illuminates the possible vicious cycle that may be trapping Elvira. We're also listening for, and testing hypotheses about, the core processes that are implicated in her suffering. Although at this point, we're not primarily intervening actively, we can certainly make tentative probes, usually in the form of Socratic questions and validation strategies, to see where the soft spots might be, and where problematic processes might not yield easily, if at all. This way of working should undermine any notions that CBT rapidly reaches for thought records or pushes people to change the way they think or behave.

In the case of Elvira, we can make the following inferences:

1. Elvira is experiencing a number of automatic thoughts, some of which may be quite accurate, rather than reflecting distortions. We might invite her to talk about how she has addressed her concern with her husband, to learn about her own perspective-taking skills and problem-solving strategies. We do know that Elvira has begun to crystalize a sense of self as trapped and helpless to deal with the challenges she is facing. So while her thoughts about her marital relationship may be accurate, her responses to them do contain potential biases and misappraisals such as "I don't deserve to stand up for myself," "I am a burden," and "I am helpless and trapped."

2. Elvira is caught in a rule-governed process with her husband, in which the rules specify what can be talked about and who has power over which decisions. We might hypothesize that she is following implicit or explicit rules about how much she is entitled to ask for what she needs, how she can relate to her husband, and to whom she can turn for social support. In exploring this further, we might find that her loss of income, from inability to work, contributes to rule governance, such as "If I'm not pulling my own weight, then I can't ask for money from my husband."

3. Self-processes in Elvira are weakened in the area of defining her needs and more forcefully asserting her wishes for contact and connection with her children and grandchildren and perhaps in more flexible and accurate perspective taking regarding others in her life.

4. She displays an acceptance of her medical status but is haunted by the fear that she will die before seeing her children and grandchildren one last time.

5. Elvira does not describe a history of prior depressive episodes, and an episode of depression appears linked to her sense of entrapment.

6. Elvira's conflict avoidance has worked over the course of her marriage, but at a cost. At this point, the cost is steep: the loss of contact with the children and grandchildren who provide a deep source of meaning and support.

7. Elvira's strengths include her long-standing love and loyalty toward her children and grandchildren who, in turn, provide emotional sustenance to her. Elvira's acceptance of her disease status suggests a deep wisdom about life. The strength and tenacity she has displayed in her long

struggle with cancer also shows determination and persistence. She has managed life's challenges and disappointments without dipping into previous depressive episodes. Finally, she is also willing to engage in therapy and to take steps forward.

8. With a provisional formulation in hand, we can focus on how the formulation leads to a treatment plan. Working collaboratively with Elvira reveals that the problem of most importance is that of increasing contact with her children and grandchildren. Her husband is not on her agenda at this time. We might explore whether she can find a way to travel to her children, or whether contact might be increased through phone calls, Skype, or FaceTime. In addition, helping Elvira deal with her children in a forthright manner about her prognosis will be important. This will help address her fears of burdening others and hopefully will lead to increased closeness at a time when her needs for closeness are greatest.

Let's take a look at a therapy vignette, to show how the previous data were generated. As the therapist presents a case formulation to Elvira, notice how she also uses GD/SQ and DBT validation strategies to deepen the relationship and clarify the formulation:

THERAPIST: Elvira, I've been asking quite a few things here, and as you know, I'm writing down some ideas as we talk. I am wondering if I could summarize what I have heard and give an idea or two about how I see things. Would that be OK?

ELVIRA: Yes. I'd like that. I am hoping you can help me figure out how to deal with this. I'm not getting anywhere on my own. I just feel like I keep sinking.

THERAPIST: OK. Sinking, and not getting anywhere on your own, right? Can you help me understand what that sinking is like for you, how it feels, and maybe what goes through your mind when you notice you're sinking?

ELVIRA: Well, I feel it in the pit of my stomach. It's just such a feeling of loneliness and fear and sadness. (Tears form in her eyes as she talks)

THERAPIST: I can see the sadness in your eyes now, Elvira. Are there some sad thoughts or maybe sad pictures and images there?

ELVIRA: I was seeing my daughter in my mind, when she was little, like my granddaughter is now. And I am missing them both. (Cries)

THERAPIST: (Notices that patient is using the present tense, which indicates that the questioning by the therapist has brought the problems into the room, emotionally) What if we could figure out some way, today and maybe tomorrow, to get you connected in a more satisfying way with your daughter and granddaughter, more regularly for now? Would that help?

ELVIRA: Yes, that'd help. I DO talk with my daughter on the phone, but not every day. I don't want to bother her or make her too sad.

THERAPIST: (Writes down the possible automatic thoughts about being a bother or inflicting pain on her daughter by virtue of patient's terminal condition) OK, here are my thoughts, and please tell me if you think I understand. If there's anything I say here that isn't exactly the way you see it, or feel it, just let me know. I want to make sure I understand the spot you're in today.

ELVIRA: OK.

THERAPIST: (Shows a diagram to patient, which she has filled out in session) It seems to me that there are a couple of things that lead to your feeling sad and helpless. One, that you may be almost ready for hospice care. But you said that dying isn't what makes you the saddest. It's the connection with your kids and grandkids that is most important. The chance to visit them maybe one last time. And two, the pain with your husband has been going on for a long time here, and he's just not understanding or supporting you right now, even your wish to take a short trip to your daughter's and son-in-law's home. Right?

ELVIRA: Yeah. That's really it.

THERAPIST: OK. You also see yourself as trapped and unable to get away on your own. I heard you say that you don't think you can use your money as a couple to take a short trip, since you're not working now. Almost like you have this rule that says "If I'm not working, I don't deserve to spend the money." (Patient nods yes) And, your husband has gotten upset with you about this, saying that it's too expensive for you to travel. (Patient again nods) So you've responded by backing away, not arguing or trying to reason with your husband, and spending a lot of time thinking and feeling sad and alone.

ELVIRA: That's about it, alright.

THERAPIST: So while I can understand why you just want peace in your home, you're left feeling stuck about what to do. And the clock's ticking, right?

ELVIRA: Right again. Yes. I feel like you understand me. What can I do?

THERAPIST: Well, what does your radar tell you here? Do you want to try to reach your husband again, to get him more on board with you? Or do you think it's best to focus on how to make either a visit to your daughter happen, or find another way to get more contact going with her, and your granddaughter?

ELVIRA: John is always going to be John. He's always like this, and I don't think he'll change. If we could find a way for me to see my daughter and her family, and maybe stay more in touch, that's what I'd like.

THERAPIST: OK. Let's see what we can do to make it happen. We can also focus on how to deal with your kids about your illness. How would that be? I know you're worried about burdening them. But from what you've told me about your kids, and your relationship to them, I think it's possible that dealing with them openly about your disease and your prognosis might bring all of you closer, just when you need that the most.

ELVIRA: That would be wonderful.

Now that a tentative formulation has been created and agreed to by both therapist and patient, the stage is set for creating interventions to help Elvira find the best option available under the circumstances. The target problem involves helping the patient achieve a sense of connection and contact with supportive people in her life, in this case her daughter, son-in-law, and grandchildren. This is now mapped out in the following case formulation, which we share with the patient and use as a basis for a treatment agreement.

Here is another example, highlighting a different set of maintaining processes. Todd Colvin is a 45-year-old married man, with two daughters, ages 16 and 12.

Problem list	
1: Stage IV disease	5: End of active treatments
2: Marital conflict	6: Wish for contact with kids/grandkids
3: Money problems/work	7:
4: Isolation	8:
Hypothesized mechanisms Long-standing marital disharmony, exacerbating effective problem solving re: wish to increase contact with children and grandchildren. Sense of self as trapped and helpless; beliefs that she is guilty or unworthy of asserting wishes; withdrawal, isolation, and rumination further dampen problem-solving efforts	
Relation of mechanisms to problems Ensnared in pattern of avoidance and rumination, Elvira withdraws from the sources of support and meaning she cherishes, deepening her sense of self as trapped and helpless, sad and angry, as she faces palliative care.	
Triggers/precipitants for current problem Resigning from her job, creating more financial burdens Learning that active treatment has ended and palliative care will begin Old pattern of marital problems exacerbated by current life situation	
Origins of mechanisms Possibly submissive since childhood and trapped in rule-governed behavior that suggests she must please others and avoid conflict at all costs (Tentative)	
Strengths Determination for years, in the face of cancer; loving and loyal mother; long and successful career, continuing through years of cancer treatments	
Treatment plan Help Elvira increase frequency and openness of contact with her children and grandchildren, either via travel or use of Skype, FaceTime, etc.	

FIGURE 4.4 Case Formulation: Elvira Mortensen

He was diagnosed with Stage II pancreatic cancer, for which he had a surgical resection. Soon thereafter, it was discovered that his cancer had spread, and was now staged as Stage IV. He has not responded to initial chemotherapy efforts and is switching to an experimental protocol in hopes of buying time.

Mr. Colvin describes depressed mood, with increasing withdrawal and isolation from others, including his family. He notes that he sometimes spends entire days in bed, facing a wall, with the lights out. He becomes irritable with his wife and daughters if they try to coax him out of the bed. His PHQ-9 reveals moderately severe depression, without suicidal ideation. In exploring with him what is occurring mentally and emotionally while he is in bed all day, he reveals the following:

> I just lay there thinking about how much I let my family down. I failed to make enough money. I don't have enough life insurance. I didn't achieve the business success that my family deserves and expected of me. I'm afraid I'm going to die and leave them all in a terrible spot. All because of me.

He notes that his mood declines as the day progresses, as he mentally and emotionally re-lives experiences in his life that confirm his diminished sense of self. He describes his days as "one long movie replay of my failed life."

He has begun to ruminate about his deceased father, a highly successful insurance executive, who he remembers saying, "You are lazy, and I'd bet you'll spend the rest of your life working at a fast food restaurant." That was a summer during which Mr. Colvin had his first job, at a Dairy Queen, after his sophomore in high school. Mr. Colvin described a searing pain as he replays this memory over and over again in his darkened bedroom. He replayed emotionally charged memories of being slighted by his mother in favor of his siblings and of being berated by his father in front of the entire family. Feelings of shame washed through him as he ruminated on his failings, trying to identify the personal defect that accounts for his being a "failure."

At the same time, Mr. Colvin said that he had enjoyed a happy marriage and strong relationships with his two daughters, who he was now convinced he had failed. When talking about his love of his family, he cried, and then turned away, saying this was too painful a topic to discuss.

Figure 4.5 shows the Vicious Cycle, formed in the first two sessions, in interviews done in Mr. Colvin's chemotherapy suite.

The immediate activating event is his sudden onset of cancer, followed by the devastating news that it has metastasized. Other factors include his financial status, especially in light of his diminished life span. We can see that his thinking and mood are increasingly depressed. He displays a number of cognitive biases: selective attention, overgeneralized thinking, reaching globally negative interpretations of self, biased memory recall. He is also becoming trapped in the processes of depressive rumination. At the level of rules and assumptions there are rules about the role of a husband and father, such as "A real man takes care of his family. I've failed to do that, so I am not worthy." Early experiences in his life may serve

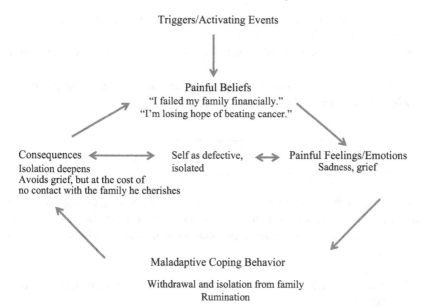

Triggers/Activating Events

Painful Beliefs
"I failed my family financially."
"I'm losing hope of beating cancer."

Consequences ⟷ Self as defective, ⟷ Painful Feelings/Emotions
Isolation deepens   isolated   Sadness, grief
Avoids grief, but at the cost of
no contact with the family he cherishes

Maladaptive Coping Behavior

Withdrawal and isolation from family
Rumination

FIGURE 4.5 Vicious Cycle: Todd Colvin

Adapted from: F. Wills (2015). *Skills in Cognitive Behaviour Therapy (2nd Edition)*. London: Sage.

as vulnerabilities to his current adaptation to cancer. He remembers his mother as having been closer to his older brother and sister and always wondered whether he had been a "mistake" late in his mother's life. He remembers his father's stinging comments, which also further bolsters his conviction that he was both a mistake and a failed disappointment to both his parents. He had struggled his entire adult life to prove himself worthy as a man.

Increasingly locked into depressive mental content and processes, he is withdrawing from the very source of love, safety, and support that has been a strength in his life. Yet he notes that to talk about this is "too painful." By turning toward the wall in his darkened bedroom, Mr. Colvin is putting his life in the service of escape and avoidance behavior. Sadly, he is thus rendered less able to move toward his most cherished source of meaning: his wife and children. Helping him move forward will, as we will see, require us to acknowledge the enormity of his suffering, bear it with him, and help him carry that pain with him while he engages with his family.

Let's turn to Mr. Colvin's self-processes. Joan Didion, the novelist and essayist, famously wrote, "We tell ourselves stories in order to live" (Didion, 2006, p. 185). Creating a sense of narrative coherence is an apparent necessity for humans, and a disruption in one's sense of meaning and in one's sense of self and world can be powerful (Frankl, 1992; Strosahl & Robinson, 2008; Hayes, Villatte, et al., 2011). Preserving one's arbitrarily constructed story of self can a source of therapy-interfering beliefs and behavior (Leahy, 2001). The "storied" self in which Todd

Colvin is caught is one of failure, unworthiness, shame, and diminishment. His depressive retreat reduces his contact with other aspects of self and with opportunities to engage with ways of being based on engagement with loved ones, even with the pain of impending loss.

Now take a moment to consider what you and Mr. Colvin might put on his problem list for therapy. Write it down:

Problem #1 _____

Problem #2 _____

Problem #3 _____

Now take a moment to consider how some of the organizing principles for our CBT model might guide our therapy, now that we have an initial case conceptualization, and you have considered possible problems toward which the therapy will be directed:

1. Normalizing Mr. Colvin's distress in the context of the challenges he is facing;
2. Creating a balance of acceptance, mindfulness, and change strategies;
3. Incorporating techniques that address cognitive *content*, in the form of cognitive biases, and cognitive *processes*, such as worry and rumination;
4. Balancing the more rationalist CBT interventions with experiential strategies;
5. Working with self-processes;
6. Working in a contextual manner to help him engage in purposeful action to access wellsprings of support and caring in his environment, despite cancer and emotional distress;
7. How the use of the therapist's self in relation to the patient can be employed to deepen the relationship and set the stage for more adaptive coping.

We will return to Mr. Colvin's case in Chapter 6. His case conceptualization form, with a treatment plan and possible barriers to care, are available in that chapter.

Let's now turn to the issue of how to create a case formulation when longer term adaptive difficulties are a part of the clinical picture. In these cases, clinicians on the team can be puzzled by, and become irritated with, seemingly self-destructive, emotionally dysregulated, and non-adherent patient behavior. The consultant in such situations needs to not only help the patient but also must help the team understand the patient. This may include addressing with the team specific strategies for managing the challenging patient. For fuller case formulations, I will adapt the formulations and worksheets created by Persons (1989; 2008), Kuyken et al. (2009), Wills & Sanders (2013), and Wills (2015).

With long-standing adaptive difficulties, we begin to build a cross-sectional analysis (Kuyken et al., 2009; J. Beck, 2011a). This lets us understand the range of situations in the patient's life in which adaptive problems manifest themselves. I've chosen to use the Vicious Cycle diagram (Figure 4.1) to map one key situation, though one can use this to map out multiple situations that spark painful emotions, cognitions, and behavior. This, in turn, can suggest that not only are there difficulties across multiple situations in life, as we might find in severe major depressive disorder, but we can begin to assess how long-standing such difficulties might be.

As we've noted, people with histories of adverse childhood events, such as abuse and neglect, can be at heightened risk of psychological and physical problems in adulthood. Knowing about adverse life histories can help the cancer team identify vulnerable patients, and it can help clinicians conceptualize the ways in which the patient's historical repertoire of responding to distress can intrude on the challenges of managing cancer in the here-and-now. It is important to emphasize that this does not mean that we are necessarily doing schema-focused or other long-term work with chronic patterns of dysfunction. We likely do not have the time, nor might the patient. But we can use our GD/SQ and validation strategies to help normalize patient behavior, for the patient and their teams, when their behavior might otherwise prove off-putting to the team. Helping patients and caregivers understand that certain treatment-interfering behaviors serve a historically valid and understandable function is freeing. It does not mean validating behaviors that are damaging. We will explore an example of this next.

The Vicious Cycle diagram is shown at the bottom of Figure 4.6, and the longitudinal factors, which contribute to the maintenance of the cycle, are speculated about, above.

In this case conceptualization, the therapist is able to hypothesize about recurrent patterns, including long-standing developmental patterns and factors. These include rules and assumptions as well as repetitive maladaptive coping strategies that the patient has employed to meet life challenges. We are also able to assess possible longitudinal factors in the person's development, which can either protect or negatively impact the person's strategies for coping. Knowing historical factors that promote resilience can help greatly in bringing patient strengths and resources to bear on the challenges of dealing with cancer. Kuyken et al. (2009) included these developmental processes as "longitudinal explanatory factors" (p. 217). These factors do not focus not only on the *events* that may have been implicated in the patient's history of suffering, but also, especially, on the person's *response* to those events. These responses include the beliefs developed about self, others, and world, or core beliefs, and also the rules, assumptions, and coping strategies by which the person attempts to deal with the world thereafter. The cycle mapped out at the bottom of the formulation shows the reciprocal, interacting processes of cognition, emotion, behavior, and consequences, activated by specific trigger situation AEs. The formulation is always a work in progress, and it is revised as new data help refine this. In addition, the formulation is a collaborative process, with the patient fully engaged in the creation and modification of the case conceptualization.

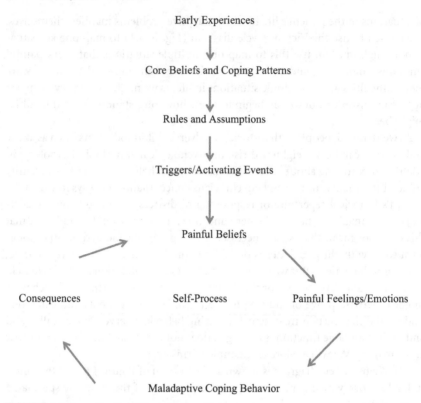

Early Experiences

Core Beliefs and Coping Patterns

Rules and Assumptions

Triggers/Activating Events

Painful Beliefs

Consequences   Self-Process   Painful Feelings/Emotions

Maladaptive Coping Behavior

FIGURE 4.6 Longitudinal Formulation Map

Adapted from: F. Wills (2015). *Skills in Cognitive Behaviour Therapy (2nd Edition)*. London: Sage.

Let's now take another case and see how the previous case conceptualization looks when it is fleshed out for a patient with long-standing adaptive difficulties. In this case, we will address the formulation for a young woman with breast cancer. She also presents with a history of childhood trauma, including long-standing substance abuse. Janice Keyes is a 23-year-old single woman, living with her boyfriend. She identified a lump in her right breast, which she ignored for months. Then she noticed another lump, in her armpit, which made it painful to lift her arm. Finally, she decided to visit a doctor, who promptly suggested the possibility of breast cancer. She was referred to the university cancer center, where a biopsy was done, confirming a Stage III metastatic breast cancer. She had hoped to have a double mastectomy, with reconstructive surgery, to provide her with the breasts she wished for—larger and, to her mind, more attractive. However, due to intense anxiety and tearfulness in a visit with her surgeon, she was referred to a psychologist. In the first session, she revealed a history of intravenous (IV) methamphetamine abuse, including during the time she had received her initial round of chemotherapy, prior to surgery. She understood that the psychologist needed to confer with the surgeon about this, as methamphetamine use might interfere with recovery from surgery. Indeed, the breast surgeon and plastic surgeon declined to pursue the mastectomy and opted for a less invasive and hence less physically taxing surgery for the patient. They offered her a lumpectomy, which left no need for reconstructive surgery. On the other hand, the surgical option did not offer the ideal protection from the spread of cancer or for recovery. The medical teams urged her to continue meeting with the psychologist and to commit to refraining from methamphetamine abuse which, in fact, she shared with her boyfriend.

The patient revealed a history of multiple adverse childhood experiences. Janice's distress tolerance was limited. She believed that the only way to handle the distress she felt, psychologically and physically in the form of intense anxious arousal, was to use drugs.

She denied being under the influence of drugs during her visits with the psychologist, but did acknowledge occasional use, including IV use, just prior to her chemotherapy infusions. She admitted to using perhaps three times a week. She expressed a strong wish to stop using drugs and recognized that it would imperil her recovery prospects, which she desired greatly.

She strongly believed that "I can't stand the emotional pain" and that "I have to use drugs to kill the pain I'm in." Interpersonally, she had few safe havens in life but identified a family who took her in while she finished high school. But there, too, her drug abuse led them to eject her immediately after high school, due to concerns about their own children. This contributed to Janice's sense that she was shameful, defective, and unlovable. She reported mental confusion and concentration and attention problems, possibly related to drug use and chemotherapy. Because she lived two hours away from the cancer center, she was housed at a free lodge for medical patients, while in the city for her cancer therapy. Here, she is alone.

She was not without strengths and important life values. One powerful motivator for her was her wish to see her father, a career military man, from whom she had been estranged for many years, and who was soon to return from a deployment in Afghanistan. Her strengths also included not only loyalty to her father, but also a decent work history, and the accrual of college credits, which she hoped would lead to a degree and a better life for her.

The case formulation highlights the current problems facing this young woman. We can see both the current factors that are maintaining her difficulties as well as the developmental factors that contributed to her tragically destructive coping strategies. The reciprocal interaction between her beliefs about self and others, her limited distress tolerance, and her coping strategy of killing pain via drugs all had painful consequences as she faced cancer. Yet her wish to live and to connect with her estranged father set the stage for the development of possible new coping strategies. The problem list will certainly include support for cessation of illicit drugs, including IV methamphetamine, during the remainder of her cancer therapy, if that is possible. This could include referral to a drug counselor and possible Narcotics Anonymous sponsor to support cessation of drugs.

The wisdom of identifying patients with histories of adverse childhood experiences is also highlighted by this case. But our focus is on the more here-and-now

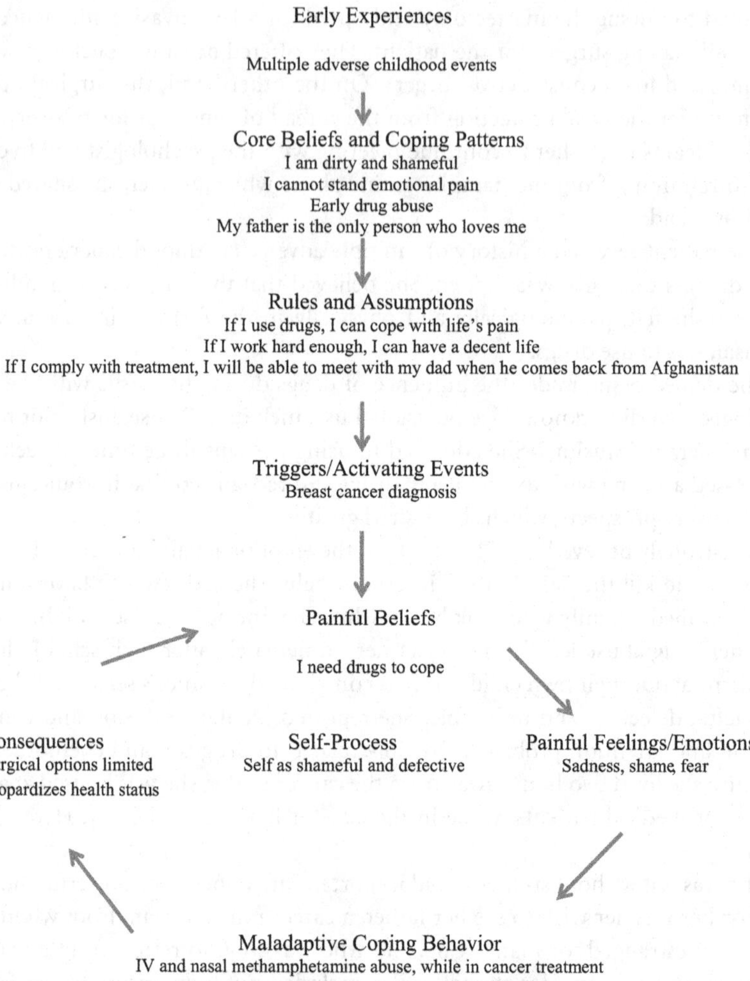

Early Experiences

Multiple adverse childhood events

↓

Core Beliefs and Coping Patterns
I am dirty and shameful
I cannot stand emotional pain
Early drug abuse
My father is the only person who loves me

↓

Rules and Assumptions
If I use drugs, I can cope with life's pain
If I work hard enough, I can have a decent life
If I comply with treatment, I will be able to meet with my dad when he comes back from Afghanistan

↓

Triggers/Activating Events
Breast cancer diagnosis

↓

Painful Beliefs

I need drugs to cope

Consequences	Self-Process	Painful Feelings/Emotions
Surgical options limited	Self as shameful and defective	Sadness, shame, fear
Jeopardizes health status		

Maladaptive Coping Behavior
IV and nasal methamphetamine abuse, while in cancer treatment

FIGURE 4.7 Longitudinal Formulation Map: Janice Keyes

Adapted from: F. Wills (2015). *Skills in Cognitive Behaviour Therapy (2nd Edition)*. London: Sage.

challenge of dealing with cancer and adhering to the demands of cancer treatment. This will require helping her find reasons to persist in adhering to difficult and frightening procedures while refraining from the drug use that she has historically employed to avoid or escape emotional pain.

Chapter Summary

Case formulations in CBT guide treatment by generating hypotheses about key problems and the factors maintaining those problems. The process of creating a formulation begins in the first session. We seek to create a formulation that fits the time limitations we may face with each patient. In some cases, a formulation that confines itself to understanding one key problem, in one circumscribed situation, is sufficient. In other cases, complexities of patient history, and dysfunctional patterns over multiple situations in the patient's life, will require a more thorough case formulation. Case formulations are always provisional and are built on testable clinical hypotheses. Formulations are subject to revision on the basis of patient input and on testing our hypotheses, in session and in homework done between sessions. Formulations set the stage for selecting treatment strategies and for guiding the direction of our therapy.

Key Points

1. A strong case formulation incorporates all relevant factors affecting the patient's presentation, beginning with the effects of cancer and its treatment. This includes the relevant cognitive, emotional, and behavioral responses to cancer, focusing on both maintain factors in the problem(s), and the patient's strengths and values.

2. Formulations begin in the first session, as we make tentative hypotheses and structure our sessions in a way that allows us to both connect with the patient(s) and clarify problems and maintaining factors.

3. Formulations are continually subject to revision, on the basis of a collaborative process between the therapy and the patient.

4. A case formulation in CBT strives to be parsimonious.

5. By setting up a collaboratively derived problem list and sharing our formulation with the patient, we set the stage for therapeutic change.

6. Case conceptualizations can be focused on one key problem, in one circumscribed situation.

7. Depending upon case complexity and time, we can assess multiple situations involved in the maintenance of patient difficulties as well as the longitudinal factors implicated in the patient's functioning.

8. CBT case formulations employ the organizing principles presented earlier to not only understand the processes in which the patient is stuck but also generate treatment strategies that target those processes for intervention.

9. It sets the stage for a change agenda, with change broadly conceptualized to include acceptance and change processes.

Part II
Clinical Applications

Five
Understanding Depression in Cancer Patients

Symptoms of depression are common signs of distress in cancer patients, though as we've seen, prevalence rates vary, for a number of reasons. First, symptoms of depression overlap with the effects of cancer and its treatments, including fatigue and sleep and appetite disturbances. Second, depression in cancer patients may present as different from depression in psychiatric settings; for example, cancer patients may present with fewer of the cognitive distortions that characterize depression in non-medically ill patients. Third, a diagnosis of depression requires patients to meet a threshold for diagnosis, using the *DSM*. Cancer patients may present with sub-syndromal depression yet have impairments in the quality of life and in adaptive functioning. Fourth, estimates may be derived from very heterogeneous treatment populations.

Li et al. (2012) questioned the accuracy of using *DSM* criteria for major depressive disorder as a means of screening for depression in cancer patients. They noted that "a majority of depressive presentations in cancer are sub-threshold and therefore may be under-recognized and untreated" (p. 1188). And if we use depressive symptoms, rather than MDD, as our criteria, up to 58% of cancer patients may report depressive symptoms (Massie, 2004). We do know, not surprisingly, that depression is more common in cancer patients than in the general population. Jacobsen and Andrykowski (2015) suggested that the best estimate comes from a recent meta-analysis by Mitchell et al., (2013), who found that 14.9% of cancer patients meet criteria for *DSM* depression. This contrasts a 12-month prevalence rate of 6.7% in the general U.S. population (Kessler et al., 2005).

Depression in cancer patients is linked to a host of problems including greater disability, increased risk of mortality, increased report of pain, increased rates of utilization of hospital-based care, and heightened risk of suicide. Vulnerability to depression includes a prior history of depression. Hill et al. (2011) found that up to 67% of cancer patients who presented with episodes of major depressive disorder were experiencing a recurrence of a previous disorder. Other contributing factors to depression include limited social support, an avoidant coping style, a family history of depression, and an increased burden of cancer symptoms. In fact, the latter, disease burden, which includes functional disability, stage of disease, and the number of physical symptoms, "is one of the strongest and most consistent predictors of depressive symptoms" (Li et al., 2012, p. 1188). Site of disease is implicated in rates of depression, with pancreatic cancer having higher rates of depression, for example.

Among the challenges of accurately diagnosing depression in cancer patients is the fact that there is overlap between the symptoms of depression and the symptoms of cancer and its treatment. For example, fatigue, anorexia, insomnia, and cognitive impairment overlap with depression (Li et al., 2012). In addition, as noted earlier, the pattern of thinking that tends to characterize depression in the general population may not be as prominent in cancer patients (Pasquini et al., 2008).

Clinicians therefore need a framework for assessing and working with depression, whether criteria for major depressive disorder are met, or whether depression is sub-syndromal and related to adjustment difficulties to cancer. The case formulation model in Chapter 4 allows for the creation of a robust and practical understanding of the patient, regardless of the presenting features, pervasiveness, duration, or severity of depression. Because we are relying on transdiagnostic processes, the formulation can be tailored to the specific presentations of each patient. In this chapter, we will briefly address the following: screening for depression; assessing for key depressive emotional, cognitive, and behavioral processes in clinical interviews; and treatment for these processes.

Rapid Screening

A broad screening instrument, such as the Edmonton Symptom Assessment System-Revised (ESAS-R; see Appendix) (Bruera & Macdonald, 1993; Chang et al., 2000; Nekolaichuk et al., 2008), allows the clinician to make a quick assessment of overall functioning and to home in on relevant areas of difficulty. Although the ESAS-R was developed for use in palliative care, it provides a quick, easy-to-use screening tool for many of the patients who present to behavioral health clinics, after an initial screening by the medical team has occurred. The form does not contain the term "palliative care" and is therefore non-threatening or stigmatizing. What it does accomplish, however, is a quick rating of many of the key areas that will become targets for our problem list. It is a point-in-time rating scale, asking about patient distress and suffering as it is being experienced in this moment. The use of additional self-report scales, such as the PHQ-9, can follow.

Besides its utility as a screening tool for depression, the PHQ-9 also directly asks about suicidality. In turn, the clinical interview can be focused on the problematic content areas that are revealed in the ESAS-R as well as the PHQ-9. It then becomes possible to separate out the relative contributions of the effects of cancer and treatment-related fatigue, pain, and sleep and appetite problems from the more depressive responses of the patient. In addition, it is possible to find evidence of prior episodes of depression as well as learning about the patient's response to previous treatment efforts. A history of depression tends to predict recurrence. Those with two or more prior episodes have a 70% to 80% likelihood of recurrence (Segal et al., 2013). Depressed cancer patients, especially those with prior episodes, should be given information about treatment options, including medication therapy. And if they responded to prior medication trials, that option should be discussed as well (including with the referring team).

In addition to looking very broadly at mood and anxiety problems, the ESAS-R also inquires about overall well-being. This dimension is of particular importance in our efforts, because we are not concerned just with removing depressive symptoms. Our therapeutic objectives in CBT are also focused on enhancing well-being, a sense of purpose, and engagement in life, to the limits of one's ability to do so. There is an emerging and robust literature which suggests the health benefits of focusing on accessing and building positive emotions, well-being, and purpose, rather than focusing solely on removing depression or anxiety symptoms, for cardiovascular disease (Nezu et al., 2005; Cohen et al., 2016) and for cancer (Carlson & Speca, 2010). A discussion of the possible biological mechanisms by which these factors influence health status is beyond the scope of this book, although research suggests a relationship between well-being, purpose, and the downregulation of chronic intense, painful emotion arousal. These factors, in turn, can influence inflammation and immune functioning (Lutgendorf & Anderson, 2015). Whether this, in turn, influences longevity is highly controversial; the focus here is on living as fully and meaningfully as possible, even with advanced disease.

A focus on acceptance, strengths, purpose, and well-being all combine to shift the CBT agenda from one of simply removing depression to that of enhancing meaningful engagement with life and having a life worth living. This broader perspective of treatment, introduced into CBT by ACT, DBT, and MBCT, adds dignity and vitality to our treatment efforts.

Clinical Guidelines: Using the Model for Understanding Depression in Cancer Patients

The following psychotherapeutic guidelines are used to assess for depression and to target problems for intervention. The organizing principles presented in Chapter 2 allow us to identify relevant processes that have gone awry, based on functional impairments and patient distress, at any level of depression, whether syndromal or sub-syndromal. As we will see in clinical applications, our primary emphasis in treatment involves building on patient strengths in a way that seeks to foster well-being, resting on a scaffolding of action directed toward engagement with life.

Working with the Patient's Depressive Emotions

CBT is most meaningful when it connects to a core of emotion, as we have seen. When patients are unable to readily identify automatic thoughts, emotion itself often provides a royal road to meaning. When the patient's responses to rating scales and affect in session suggest distress, we invite the patient to access, experience, and put words to their emotions. Besides rating scales, the patient's body and affect often convey states of sadness, defeat, hopelessness, and entrapment. Patients' families are often alarm bell ringers, noticing disturbing changes related to cancer and depressive emotion, depressed thinking, and depressive behavior. Consistent with our emphasis on normalizing distress, our first step might be to open the door to painful, distressing emotions by gently inviting the patient's emotions into the room and then normalizing them. By doing so, we provide psychoeducation about the role of emotions as signals and as calls to action, not as internal enemies. In this way, psychoeducation is not just a dry exercise in giving information. Done properly, psychoeducation becomes a way to introduce acceptance and for distancing from problematic cognitive content and processes. The therapist strives to refrain from becoming too wordy or from attempts to overpower emotions with cognitions (Wills & Sanders, 2013). A list of possible questions and statements to elicit and foster emotion expression includes:

1. Validation, to support the patient in accepting their emotions as valid in context. Questions here might include, "If sadness is a signal, what is it telling you right now?"

2. Clarifying primary and secondary emotions (Greenberg, 2011; Koerner, 2012), by asking questions such as "Is this the rock bottom emotion you are feeling?" and "Is there another emotion lurking below the emotion you have talked about so far?" (Wills & Sanders, 2013).

3. Adopting an accepting and compassionate therapeutic posture, including appropriate therapeutic silence. Leahy (2001) described the importance of "weeping for the plague," which we must balance with our need to also foster active coping and engagement strategies. In this sense, emotional pain itself is not a problem, unless it becomes entailed with avoidance or entanglement in cognitive and behavioral processes that stoke depression or anxiety. We also model compassion, which we invite the patient to experience toward self (Gilbert, 2009a; Hayes, 2016).

4. Exploring for signs of experiential avoidance, including avoidance of emotions, which is a transdiagnostic factor in psychological disorders (Harvey et al., 2004; Hayes, Villatte et al., 2011), and for cancer patients,

specifically (Stanton et al., 2015). We must be mindful of the patient who is walled off from experiencing or expressing emotions, even when those emotions are adaptive bearers of life's messages. Walling off emotions or the expression of emotions can be driven by rules such as "If I cry, I'm weak," "I mustn't trouble others," "My emotions will overwhelm others," or "I have to be strong for my wife and children." Metacognitive beliefs such as "It is dangerous to feel strong feelings" or "If I feel sad, I'll make my cancer worse" may lie behind emotion avoidance as well.

The therapist's open, accepting stance toward inner experience may cue the patient to access and express emotions and thoughts in a safe environment. Paradoxically, allowing emotions to be present, without struggling against them, can help regulate emotions and reduce their intensity. This can allow for a more flexible, adaptive re-working of the meaning of illness and for the development of fresh strategies for coping. A clean experience of emotional pain would be sadness, grief, and raw fear at the prospect of facing a life-altering and potentially life-threatening disease. The emotion here serves as a signal for possible losses and threats and may well be quite logical and appropriate to the context. As Teasdale and Chaskalson (2011a, b) and Hayes, Villatte et al. (2011) noted, drawing on Buddhist spiritual traditions, clean emotional pain differs from suffering. When emotional pain becomes entailed with non-acceptance and fusion with seemingly out-of-control and unwanted cognitive content and cognitive processes it becomes suffering. Linehan noted that pain + non-acceptance = suffering, and that "the way out of suffering is through Radical Acceptance" (Linehan, 2015, p. 459).

The patient's ability to tolerate and deal with emotional distress can simply be swamped by the impact of cancer in a human life. For example, reviewing the patient's history of managing prior challenges in life can help determine whether a focus on distress tolerance might be needed. A key task for the clinician working with cancer patients is to determine when and how to bring emotional pain into the room and when to respect the patient's need or wish to avoid experiencing and expressing intense emotion. Loss and grief are common companions in cancer-related depression, for example.

Tracking the Link between Depression and the Physical Effects of Cancer and Cancer Therapies

It is important to learn about the physical consequences of cancer and cancer therapy, including pain and fatigue. These effects can cue depression, including losses of key roles, the breakdown in daily routines, loss of access to positive experiences, and what Strosahl and Robinson (2008) referred to as "depression compression," the shrinking life space associated with depression. This accrual of losses in daily activities can compound to affect the patient's sense of self and become represented in their appraisals of self, others, and world. Steps to utilize activity scheduling or Behavioral Activation have to be balanced with an understanding of cancer-related pain and fatigue. Only then can we begin to assess the ability and the willingness of the patient to push toward increased activity levels.

Cognitive Content and Cognitive Processes in Cancer-Related Depression

One key avenue for understanding depression in cancer patients is to access and explore the cognitive content and processes that may be fueling depressive emotion and behavior (Moorey & Greer, 2012). This includes assessing not only for the presence of Beck's Cognitive Triad (A. Beck & Rush, 1979) but also beliefs related to one's ability to navigate challenges. A view of self as trapped, helpless, and overwhelmed can impair problem-solving abilities (Nezu et al., 1999; Nezu et al., 2007; Nezu et al., 2012). It is important to recognize that not all mood-driven and dysphoric reflection is necessarily a sign of depression. A rapid onset of a serious health threat can spark a life review that sometimes veers into painful directions (Yalom, 1980). The process of benefit finding in cancer, the teachable moments that cancer can provide, often emerge only after making contact with the painful consequences of earlier decisions: relationships unattended to, people harmed by acts of omission and commission, roads in life not taken, talents not cultivated, decisions regretted only with the benefit of hindsight. Such concerns in and of themselves are not necessarily indicative of depression. Depressive reflection, when coupled with deepening dysphoria, selective attention, depressive memory biases, withdrawal and isolation, can the stage can be set for another toxic cognitive *process*: rumination.

Biases in Cognitive Content

Cognitive biases in depression can fuel suffering, as identified in Beck's Cognitive Triad (A. Beck & Rush, 1979) as well as other cognitive biases that may contribute to depression (Harvey et al., 2004). Cognitive biases in the Cognitive Triad include global and invalidating beliefs about self, about one's expectations of others and the world, and about the future. *All-or-none thinking* can include beliefs such as "If I can't do everything I used to do, then I am worthless." *Overgeneralization* can include beliefs such as "Because I couldn't go to my kids' soccer game last night, I'm not much of a mom." *Mind reading* can include "All my co-workers think I'm a freak." *Fortune-telling* may involve "Because I'm so tired, I will never be able to live my life again." *Discounting the positive* can include "I made cookies last night for my kids; but so what? I couldn't make dinner." *Self-labeling* might include "I'm a failure as a father."

In working with cancer patients, we want to be careful to assess the patient's understanding of their disease state, and match it with the appraisals of their oncology team, before assuming that biases or distortions are present. For example, a 36-year-old woman with Stage I breast cancer was successfully treated and told at her first follow-up visit that she had excellent recovery and survival prospects. When asked about how that information was being received, she said, "If there's a 90% chance that I'll survive past 5 years, it means there's a 10% chance I won't. I *know* I'll be in that 10%."

Depressive cognitive content can reveal itself in the form of beliefs such as "I'm letting everyone down," "I did something to deserve this," and "No matter what my doctor says, I know I'm going to die from this." Other forms of cognitive bias can include the recency effect, such that patients assume that the sickness and fatigue they experience during chemotherapy will extend into the future: "Since I have felt sick this past 2 months, it will always be like this," or the reverse belief, "I shouldn't be feeling sick; it's been 2 months, and I should be over this." Selective attention, another transdiagnostic factor in psychological disorders, can show up in the form of hyperattunement to cancer-related information, available online, on television, followed by personalizing and interpreting that information in a catastrophic light. Similarly, selective attention to bodily sensations, including pain, fatigue, and sensations from surgical scars or radiation therapy, interpreted in a catastrophic way, can form a bedrock for both depression and anxiety.

Rigid and inflexible rules can also be implicated in non-acceptance and in depression. Williams, M. et al. (2015) and Segal et al. (2013) described one key contributing factor to depression, in terms of the gap between how things are in one's life, and how one wishes or expects things to be in one's life. Linehan has noted that in challenging situations, one can fix the problem, one can change one's emotional response to the problem, one can accept the problem, or one can stay miserable. "This should not be happening to me," "I should be better by now," "I can't live with my appearance," and "I'm not supposed to be this tired" are all examples of implicit rules, whose violation by cancer and treatment may fuel non-acceptance and ineffective problem-solving strategies.

As a rule, when significant cognitive biases are present, the therapist is well advised to address cognition before trying other avenues of intervention. The range of intervention strategies includes the more rationalist approaches designed by Beck, the more experiential approaches found in ACT, mindfulness and acceptance-based strategies for cognition, and psychoeducational approaches regarding how minds work, outlined as follows. All are designed to help create distance on stuck thinking, in multiple modes of information processing, to allow more flexible engagement in managing and/or solving problems.

Rumination

As noted in Chapter 2, rumination is a cognitive *process* that serves as a key risk factor for depression recurrence and is a key maintaining factor for a current episode of depression. Standard CBT techniques intended to address biased and/or problematic cognitive *content* may fail when addressing rumination, since it is the process itself that is toxic. Once entering a cycle of rumination, not only is global behavior affected but also one's problem-solving skills are affected adversely (Harvey et al., 2004). Inviting discussion of how the patient is handling sad mood and bad news can quickly reveal whether rumination is encroaching on mood and daily functioning, using prompts such as "Tell me what's going through your mind during times when you are sitting alone, inwardly focused." Patterns of painful memory, themes of loss, diminishment, hopelessness, depressive mental imagery, painful cognitive content, and a physical posture of defeat and helplessness are all elicited in the interview. To determine if the patient is becoming trapped in a cycle of rumination and withdrawal, it is useful to ask about how much time is spent in an isolated manner, with one inadvertently marinating in depressive emotions, memories, and cognitive processes, including imagery and body sensations. Literally asking for the amount of time, or the percent of time, spent each day ruminating can be highly revealing. If a spouse or other family member is present, it can be useful to gently elicit estimates from family members, as there may well be a disparity between the family's appraisals and the patient's appraisals.

Rumination is not merely a cognitive process; it is a link in a chain of depressive behaviors, all of which unfolds in the context of the patient's ecosystem. As such, rumination involves loss of contact with the present moment and becomes part of a broader pattern of disengagement and withdrawal from life and an increasingly limited repertoire of effective problem-solving strategies. We can normalize this disengagement and withdrawal process in light of its possible evolutionary functions. As such, it may serve as a strategy to rest and restore oneself, following a perceived or impending loss or defeat (Gilbert, 2009a), which cancer can potentially represent. We also highlight the downside effects of rumination. As we will see, intervention strategies for cognitive *processes* gone awry differ from those applied to biased cognitive *content*.

Depressive Self-Processes

The physical and behavioral changes brought on by cancer can lead not only to a compressed life but also to a sense of self as trapped, diminished, helpless, and hopeless. Themes of being trapped are often characteristic of depression (Gilbert, 2009b). A self viewed as trapped, damaged, defective, and/or diminished can quickly fuel rumination, stalled problem-solving abilities, hopelessness, and suicidality.

Beck's ideas about modes of mind (A. Beck, 1996; A. Beck & Haigh, 2014) touched on self-processes. But the work of Steve Hayes brought self-processes back to a position of greater prominence in American clinical psychology (Hayes, 1984; Hayes et al., 2012) through perspective-taking skills and creating more flexible, compassionate, and wise states or processes. This, too, dovetails with MBCT (Teasdale, 1999; Segal et al., 2013), which posits modes of mind, or modes of being.

One is tempted to speak of the self as though it were a static entity or thing, which it is not. In fact, and in line with William James's early writings on this

(James, 1890), there are multiple selves, or self-states/self-processes. This, too, has been recognized in Hayes's work (Hayes, Villatte et al., 2011; Villatte et al., 2016). Self-processes are lived experiences, composed of verbal and emotional processes, body sensations, and action urges. It is a place to stand from which one views and deals with the world (Hayes, 2016). The limit of words to fully describe these processes speaks to the need to foster experiences in session to help the depressed patient access such processes. The capacity to flexibly access more adaptive self-states, or self-processes, offers a potential pathway out of depression and into a greater state of well-being, regardless of circumstances. DBT's insistence that all are wise and possess the capacity for Wise Mind, too, is an acknowledgment that humans experience multiple self-states, the accessing of which can free or entrap a human life. Within the more Beckian tradition, newer work by Bennett-Levy et al. (2015) focused on helping people build new states of being, or self-states, not as a means of removing or extinguishing older, less functional self-states, but as competing memory representations, capable of showing up purposefully and with increased frequency in a person's life. Thus, CBT for cancer-related depression can perhaps gain added power by working with the thinker, the experiencing and doing self, not just the thoughts.

The ability to make sense of experience is a fundamental human capability and need. The loss of one's sense of narrative coherence, and hence one's sense of self, is immensely unsettling, sparking potentially depressive and/or anxious processes, unless or until a fresh experience of narrative coherence is achieved. A sense of purpose and meaning can enhance not only quality of life but also mortality rates (Frankl, 1986; 1992; Cohen et al., 2016). Its loss can be devastating. In turn, thera-peutic efforts can be directed toward helping patients rework a functional and vital sense of meaning and purpose: a sense of self as capable of meeting challenges.

One of the reasons that benefit finding may occur in cancer patients is that the threat to self, occasioned by a diagnosis of cancer, may also set the stage for a renewed, more flexible, wise, and compassionate sense of self. Whether these self-states are temporary or become part of a new repertoire that is continually built over the course of one's remaining life is doubtless dependent upon many factors, but facilitating these self-processes and the growth of behavioral repertoires that support them is a key offering that behavioral health can potentially make in can-cer therapy.

Mindfulness Processes in Depression

MBCT, DBT, and ACT all foster present moment processes, including the capacity to step back from the stream of mental events and into this moment. The capac-ity to enter this moment simultaneously involves multiple other processes: accep-tance shows up when entering the present moment, in the form of acceptance of emotions, body sensations, and thoughts; awareness of non-cancer areas of a human life can open up; the capacity to observe, notice, and choose can be fos-tered in the present moment. Mindfulness often means relaxation, or zoning out, to people, especially those who have no cultural or personal experience of mindfulness as a discipline. Mindfulness is not about either zoning out or relaxing. Although some patients find mindfulness exercises to be peaceful, our intent is not to induce peace through avoidance. Mindfulness processes are fostered in CBT through experiential interventions. Rather, practices of this sort may foster a sense of being able to settle, be present, notice, and observe experience from a place of safety. In addition, the interpersonal context of therapy, can foster a sense of safety and compassion. The therapist is always present, to the patient, to the process, and to the shared endeavor of helping to access resources to ease suffering. For highly distressed patients, who have histories of difficulty tolerating distress, it is wise and necessary to avoid immersion in internal processes that may swamp the patient's coping reserves. This is important for both depression and anxiety treatment. In fact, when distress tolerance is low, distress is high, and time is a key factor, there is an important place for pharmacotherapy, either instead of or in addition to mindfulness and acceptance work with cancer patients.

With respect to rumination, as well as worry, the antidote is found in the present moment. Suspension of depressive rumination is a treatment target for depression and includes the fostering of mindfulness and acceptance processes as well as active contact and engagement with the ongoing contexts of daily life.

A Focus on Strengths, Resources, and Values

Depression brings with it a loss of contact with or at least a muting of effective contact with adaptive strengths, emotional support, interpersonal contact, and engagement in actions that reflect one's deepest values, one's true north. During the assessment and formulation process, the therapist explores areas of strength and meaning in sufficient detail to generate hypotheses about how therapy can be organized around re-engagement. This begins with the process of joining, in the first session. Rather than focusing solely on removing the symptoms of depression, the energy for therapy comes from helping people contact important facets of their lives that cancer and depression have affected and to reclaim those areas as much as possible. More flexible cognitive and behavioral responses can then be accessed to create self-sustaining patterns of behavior that lead to a virtuous cycle out of depression.

Contextual Work with Depression: Dealing with Life Engagement Strategies

CBT involves not only addressing internal processes but also increasing meaningful engagement with the process of living, through action. As a general rule, we don't ask the patient to change behavior until we have an understanding of what is maintaining their difficulties in the first place. Understand first, go for a change agenda next. CBT is rooted in behavior therapy, and behavior change, including a balance of acceptance and change, is very much a part of brief work with cancer patients. So, too, a broader understanding of the patient's relationship to his or her ecosystems, including family, friends, co-workers, spiritual communities, the medical teams, and others, is vital in putting an action plan together. The purpose of the action plan is to help the patient engage in broader, self-sustaining interactions with sources of strength, and meaning, ideally in multiple contexts of daily life. Helping people make experiential contact with what matters most in their life can set the stage for bringing behavior in line with those values. Thus, the ruminator who escapes the pain of his losses by turning to the wall can also see that the price of facing the wall is the loss of contact with loved ones. Small steps toward facing away from the real or metaphorical wall and toward life can be made with cancer patients utilizing problem-solving (Nezu et al., 1999; Nezu et al., 2007; Nezu et al., 2012) and behavioral activation (Hopko et al., 2003; Hopko et al., 2008; Hopko et al., 2011).

Choosing Treatment Modalities

Our focus will be on Cognitive Behavioral approaches to treating depression. However, medication therapy can play an important role in treatment. When the patient has a prior history of depression and/or has responded to medication therapy in the past, an assessment for anti-depressant medication is warranted. In addition, patient preference for either medication or psychotherapy, or a combination, must be taken into account and respected, before embarking on a course of treatment. The wise and ethical move is to present the evidence for the efficacy of various treatment options, explore the pros and cons, and collaborate with the patient in their selection of a treatment.

Key Points

1. The prevalence of depression in cancer patients is significantly higher than in non-cancer patients.
2. Diagnostic challenges for depression in cancer patients include the overlap between the effects of cancer and cancer therapy and the indicators of depression.
3. In addition, selecting criteria for inclusion of patients as depressed contributes to uncertainties in regards to prevalence of depression in cancer patients.
4. It is best to focus on depression in both its syndromal and sub-syndromal presentations, including a format for working with patients who may meet criteria for major depressive disorder and those whose depression is likely an adjustment problem.
5. Quick and inexpensive screeners include the Edmonton Symptom Assessment System-Revised (ESAS-R) and the PHQ-9.

6. The clinician and patient must collaborate in selecting a treatment modality, including medication therapy and/or psychotherapy for depression.

7. Clinical guidelines for each of the key processes used in the book were presented, for working with depressed cancer patients.

Six
Interventions for Depression in Cancer Patients

Think of the principles that guide this treatment model as akin to colors on the palette of a skilled painter. In a principle-based treatment, such as this, the therapist is able to mix colors from the palette in order to achieve an intended effect, depending upon the case formulation, the problem list, and the needs of the patient. By contrast, highly manualized treatment protocols may at first blush appear to be like a paint-by-number painting. Using principle-based treatments in CBT requires considerable skill and considerable judgment, thus allowing for the kind of creativity and disciplined spontaneity of a jazz musician, to switch artistic metaphors. We will focus on using the eight organizing principles outlined in Chapter 2 in our treatment of depression in cancer patients. While I will provide guidelines for selecting principles and intervention strategies, our interventions are only correct when they are accepted and useful for the patient. We rarely know in advance how an intervention will be received.

It is wise to focus on maintaining a spirit of collaboration and engagement, putting the relationship front and center at all times. If therapy drifts too far in the direction of change for the patient to tolerate or pursue, come back to the present moment, make contact with the patient, and regroup. The central dialectic observed in DBT between acceptance and change is very salient in work with cancer patients. The focus on present moment processes provides an anchor to which therapist and patient can return when needed (Wilson & DuFrene, 2009). This creates a relationship and a present moment matrix from which principles involving cognitive and behavior change and the fostering of strength-based self-processes can be cultivated. The therapist then selects strategies best suited to address the maintaining factors of patient suffering.

Interventions for Depressed Cognitive Content

The use of Beck's Guided Discovery and Socratic Questioning allows us to set the stage for people to make contact with both the nature of their beliefs and the impact of those beliefs. Then, we encourage the patient to consider whether there might be another way of viewing self and circumstances that can lead to a more adaptive outcome. Wills (2015) noted that Beckian cognitive restructuring techniques were envisioned as a three-step process: identify automatic thoughts, evaluate them, and respond to them. These steps can be rushed in ways that back-fire, by promoting patient resistance, damaging the therapeutic alliance, and inad-vertently deepening patient entanglement in painful beliefs. The CBT therapist is wise to remember that cognitive change is not eliminative. We are not trying to get rid of the bad thoughts and have only good thoughts. We are helping create flexible alternatives that are more functional and that are available in emotionally charged circumstances. Combining Guided Discovery with Validation techniques allows for a softer stance toward engaging with patient beliefs, especially those that are entrenched and/or emotionally compelling to the patient. A rough hierarchy of techniques for addressing problematic cognitive content is as follows:

1. Soft probes of beliefs: no challenges of the validity of beliefs, while fos-tering compassion toward self;
2. Mind education: gentle psychoeducation about how minds work;
3. Evidence searching;
4. Searching for possible disconfirming evidence;
5. Creating functional alternative explanations;
6. Exploring the function of living as though a belief is true/false;
7. Metaphor and experiential exercises;
8. Mindfulness of thoughts, letting go of the stream of thought;
9. Perspective-taking and self-process work.

This hierarchy is offered tentatively, and I would advise experienced clinicians to experiment with this. For example, I place mindfulness and perspective-taking interventions at the bottom of the list. Other CBT treatment models might place them far higher up on the list for early interventions, to wit: ACT and MBCT. A simple, common sense focus in this hierarchy may comport with the needs of patients who in many cases have never seen a behavioral health professional. There is no one intervention that will generally work for all patients and no clear order of intervening. Clinical work at its best is experimental: we provide a rationale for our work, including available evidence and its limitations; we assess the effective-ness of an intervention by studying its impact. If it fails, we adjust. We rectify any breaches in the treatment relationship that may occur when a strategy or interven-tion fails. We try something new.

Let's turn to a case example, to show how these interventions can be employed to good effect.

Case Example

Sally Klipsten is a 61-year-old mother of five and a grandmother of 10. She has been married to the same man for 39 years and recently learned what she described as "the worst news in the world." Her pancreatic cancer has metastasized, and any available options are both experimental and unlikely to do more than extend her life by weeks or, at most, a few months. She is despondent. She is withdrawn, and she is uncharacteristically hopeless, according to her husband, Merle, who owns and operates a small town agricultural supply company. His fear of seeing his wife retreat and give up led him to request a consultation. She has no prior history of depression. In the first session, the therapist met conjointly with the couple. Sally presented as tearful and acknowledged being depressed since learning that her Stage IV cancer was likely to end her life. In exploring the beliefs that accompanied her tears and depression, she revealed these thoughts: "I'm done," "I've let everybody down," "My grandchildren aren't going to remember me." Earlier in session, the therapist's focus was on compassionately being with the couple in the fear, sadness, and loss that Sally and Merle both face, each in their own ways.

There is no prior history of depression. So it is likely that the beliefs described previously are recent and are a response to the devastating news that Sally received. We might posit that using softer touch Beckian techniques can help her step back from these beliefs and see them in a fresh light. Then, we might find alternatives that can be linked to a behavior change strategy that brings her back into her life and out of retreat or compression mode.

THERAPIST: Sally, if I might, I'd like to go back to a couple of things you said a little while ago. You said "I'm done." May I ask what that means to you? (The therapist had asked previously how the patient prefers to be addressed)

SALLY: It means I'm going to die of this disease.

THERAPIST: Does that mean to you that you have no time left at all?

SALLY: (Thinks silently) I guess I don't know. I didn't want to ask Dr. X about that. I don't want to know.

THERAPIST: OK. And yet, it sounds as though you're assuming, when you say to yourself "I'm done," that you have *no* time.

SALLY: It feels like that. No time.

THERAPIST: Might you have many months? Maybe even more? (Therapist introduces an alternative possibility)

SALLY: I guess I don't really know. My doctor thinks I might, yes.

THERAPIST: OK. Let's say you do you have some time and some opportunities to live more fully as you wish. Would *that* matter, as far as maybe using the time you have in a way that would really matter to you and to others in your life?

SALLY: (Nods yes) It *would*.

THERAPIST: Could we take a moment to just settle in to the possibility that you have time, meaningful time ahead of you? Maybe just sit for a moment with the idea that there is some time here. (Pauses) (The therapist fosters a mindful, present moment pause for reflection)

SALLY: *Any* time would matter to me right now. (Patient sits up from previous slumped, defeated posture and makes eye contact with therapist. Her husband takes her hand)

THERAPIST: I noticed that you sat up and looked at me just now, instead of looking away. I am wondering what happened. Did you notice any differences, maybe in your emotions or your body, between "I have no time" and "I have meaningful time"? (Therapist helps patient discriminate between mood and body consequences of two differing ways of looking at the time she has)

SALLY: "I have time" feels better.

THERAPIST: Feels better in what way?

SALLY: Less sad. More time to look forward to, to spend with my husband, my children, my grandchildren.

THERAPIST: And does that seem like a real possibility? (Therapist asks patient to assess plausibility of the alternative)

SALLY: I think from what my doctor said, yes, it is. (Husband states that the oncologist does not believe death is imminent, and there may be many months or another year)

THERAPIST: OK. I'm putting this together with something else you said, which was "I've let everybody down." Do you mean your family? (Patient nods yes, while husband shakes head no) May I ask what leads you to conclude that you've let the family down?

SALLY: I got sick with this disease. Now they're all worried about *me*, instead of focusing on their *own* lives. And if I can't be the grandmother I wanted to be, especially since I've been hoping to retire and be more involved, then I'm letting them all down. (Cries) They're so young, some of them. I won't be there for their sports events, their graduations, or their weddings. (Husband reaches over and touches her arm.)

THERAPIST: (Expresses genuine acknowledgment and recognition of the pain of this long-term prediction being accurate. Then, she addresses the belief that by having cancer the patient has let people down.). Sally, I can see the pain not only on your face, but on your husband's right now. May I ask you something here? I think of letting people down if I don't keep a promise, or follow through on a commitment for some reason, especially when it's of my own choosing. Did you choose to do this, to yourself or others, getting cancer? (Therapist risks using some lighthearted irreverence, sensing that the patient might respond)

SALLY: My no! (She and her husband laugh)

THERAPIST: So maybe, could we say that cancer let you all down, especially *you* right now? What if it's the cancer that's the culprit, and not you? (Therapist introduces a reframe)

SALLY: I see what you mean. And it makes sense.

In this previous vignette, several steps were taken regarding painful beliefs:

1.   The therapist explored not only evidence but possible alternatives to believing that the patient's death is imminent.
2.   A believable and seemingly realistic possibility of more time is created.
3.   The therapist encourages the patient to pause in the moment, to notice, experientially, the effects of the two beliefs, and to reinforce not only the truth of "I have more time" but its effects experientially.
4.   The therapist next helped reframe the belief that the patient had let down her family by developing cancer.
5.   A more credible and functional belief was introduced: "It was the cancer that let everyone down."
6.   The therapist focused then on the question of whether she would be remembered by her grandchildren. This evoked sadness and grief. However, sadness and grief at the prospect of dying and leaving loved ones behind is essentially clean pain; suffering comes from the compounding effects of self-blame and the belief that one will be forgotten by those left alive.
7.   This led to some specific value-based behavioral interventions that will be discussed in a later section, on pairing behavioral activation with one's chosen values and purposes in life.

Guided Discovery in this vignette does not mean a passive therapist. The therapist in this dialogue was an active agent in suggesting possible alternative ways of looking at the situation and used humor and irreverence, even in a grim situation. The key is to be collaborative and to tune in to the patient's response to interventions. The patient stated, when feedback was sought at the end of the session, that what had been most helpful in session was realizing that she was not at fault, and was not letting down her loved ones by having a Stage IV cancer.

Checking for Openness to Disconfirming Evidence

We certainly could have employed the more directive Beckian techniques, such as writing the thoughts on a white board, asking for evidence for and against the beliefs, rating believability, creating an alternative belief, and rating the believability of her painful thought at the end of the intervention. This is standard, mainstream Beckian CBT, and when it works it is quite powerful, including with cancer patients (Moorey & Greer, 2012). Since many of our patients in cancer centers have no prior experience of psychotherapy, and may have no prior experience of depression, I advise a softer entry into this process, such as demonstrated earlier. The advantage of patients having a limited prior history of depression is that biased cognitions have short roots in the soil of distress and can often be recognized rather quickly and easily for what they are, and in a light manner that does not spark a reaction against the therapist. It is important to recognize that cognitive biases are ubiquitous (Kahneman, 2011). This acknowledgment comports with our efforts to normalize cognitive biases in times of distress.

A strategy for a user-friendly check-in to determine openness to disconfirming evidence follows. One can use the strategy of "how the mind works" to help people recognize that certain cognitive biases are ubiquitous, such as the recency effect, or other biases. This may soften a potential blow that the patient might experience to what might otherwise feel like an assault on self. Sometimes depression has deeper roots, linked to long-standing beliefs about self, arising in the context of earlier phases of development.

Here is a brief dialogue that illustrates the principles in action. For that, let's return to the case of Todd Colvin, the 45-year-old man with metastatic pancreatic cancer, whose case formulation we reviewed in Chapter 4. He believes he is a failure because he has not provided for his family's future as well as he wishes he had done. In addition, he confirms this belief by remembering denigrating comments about his laziness by his father, when Todd was an adolescent.

THERAPIST: Todd, it actually pains me a bit to hear you blame yourself for any financial troubles your family may find itself in. May I ask what makes you so upset with yourself about this?

TODD: I should have saved more money. I should have gotten life insurance. I should never have taken out such a big mortgage. I should have built more retirement assets. I failed. Just like my dad said I would, years ago.

THERAPIST: Todd, are you open to my asking a bit more about this, to see if I might help find a new way to view and deal with this painful situation?

TODD: I'm open, but I'm really upset with myself.

THERAPIST: I understand. Well, here's a question. At 45, what were you thinking, about mortgages, retirement assets, and insurance?

TODD: That I had all the time in the world.

THERAPIST: Yes. All the time in the world. Just like your friends and your business colleagues assume they have, I'm guessing?

TODD: Yeah. Nobody thinks this will ever happen to them.

THERAPIST: Yeah. So you were just planning your life the best way you could, it seems. Like anyone your age might do. So if you had a crystal ball, and could have seen the future, you'd have put money away, and focused on insurance instead of on building the business?

TODD: I would. (Looks at therapist) I sure would have. (Maintains eye contact, with tears forming in his eyes)

THERAPIST: Todd, it sounds to me like you did everything you could, short of being able to read the future. Short of having that crystal ball that none of us owns.

TODD: Well, when you put it like that, I don't have one of those. I never did. Nobody does.

THERAPIST: I wish I had one, too. Without a crystal ball, though, we make the best decisions we can at the time, without knowing what the future will hold. Then, later, when the facts have come in about the decision, sometimes we can get upset with ourselves, as if we could have known then how things would turn out years later. That can be an unfair trick our minds play on us, blaming ourselves for something we couldn't have possibly known or predicted, given the facts at the time. My mind does that, too, sometimes. I've just tried to get wise to my mind's tricks.

TODD: I think I get what you mean. But still, now my family really *will* be in a jam. And it brings up such a feeling of failure, like all the things my dad said about me being lazy were true after all.

THERAPIST: Those memories of painful experiences, especially comments like your dad's can sting forever, can't they? (Patient nods) If it were your son, in the spot you were in as a kid, would you call him a failure? Lazy?

TODD: Oh, hell no. Never. My dad was a hard ass and a hard case. I tried. I tried hard. And my son helps out at home, too. I'd never say anything to my son like my father did to me.

THERAPIST: Do you deserve the same compassion you'd give to your son? If dad was a hard ass, maybe he was wrong about you. Since he's gone, who's keeping this thing going inside you?

TODD: (Silent)I guess I am. I never thought of it that way. (Makes eye contact with therapist) If I were to let go of my dad's nasty comments about me, I'm still in a helluva jam, though.

(We will come back to other ways of softening the impact of long-standing painful beliefs, dating to earlier times in development, by working with self-processes and perspective-taking skills)

THERAPIST: At least for now, does it seem that the evidence might suggest that you did your best, given the fact that you had no way of anticipating this illness? (Patient nods) OK. What if we could focus some efforts on working with you and your wife about how to plan for the future, financially? Want to consider that?

TODD: Yeah. Without a crystal ball, I did what most of the guys I know did. I built a business, took on debt, and decided I had time to build retirement assets later, after the money was rolling in. My wife and I are starting to talk about how to deal with this. She's thinking of going back and finishing school, so she'll have a career. That gives me a little more peace.

We saw that perhaps an opening occurred in Todd's willingness to consider, even briefly, that there might be an alternative explanation for his sense of failure. Importantly, Todd's early life history of his father's stinging comments strengthened his conviction that he has failed. Depressive memory, selecting mood congruent content, reinforced Todd's cognitive biases (Teasdale & Chaskalson, 2011b). The therapist set the stage by attempting to soften painful beliefs of two kinds: current beliefs that the patient had failed as a man, and a link to an old belief from childhood, stoked by memories of his father's voice. We will return to this case to describe other sets of interventions that flow from this more distanced, or defused, stance toward these beliefs: self and perspective-taking interventions as well as behavioral activation and problem-solving interventions.

My own rule of thumb for delivering Beckian CBT interventions with cancer patients is to begin with the softer style of delivery of these interventions, presented earlier. These involve maintaining a collaborative and dialogical process, with techniques that flow more gently within the context of a conversation. And in the context of a collaborative relationship, the therapist, too, is free to introduce alternative possibilities. There is a huge array of Beckian cognitive techniques, to which the interested reader is referred, available for work with cancer patients (Leahy et al., 2011; Moorey & Greer, 2012; Westbrook et al., 2012; Wills & Sanders, 2013; Greenberger & Padesky, 2015; Wills, 2015).

Education about How Minds Work

Many people may take it for granted that thoughts are to be taken seriously, painful emotions must signify that something is wrong, and automatic pilot is the only mode of operation (Kabat-Zinn, 2013; Segal et al., 2013). A little lighthearted education about how minds work can sometimes help people step back from bought thoughts and see them as just thoughts, with no compelling claim on the truth or on the person's behavior. CBT traditionally has a screening process and a process of socializing patients to the model as a condition of entering treatment. For patients in cancer centers, this may represent the first meeting in their life with a behavioral health professional, and to quickly or aggressively push against their beliefs may feel odd and off-putting. As per the guidelines in Chapter 3, we start with validation and Guided Discovery, and then look for change strategies. Psychoeducation about how the mind works can provide patients who are naïve to psychotherapy with a gentle, user-friendly walking tour of how minds work, all minds, including the therapist's. This comports with our objective of normalizing distress and suffering in the context of a severe health threat.

A sample script for this, in this case with Sally Klipsten, might go this way:

> You know, all our minds do interesting things, without our asking them to. In this case, it sounds like your mind jumped to the very painful conclusions that you're going to die fast, be forgotten, and that between now and then you've

let down your family. (Patient acknowledges this) Now your mind did this because it's trying to make sense of your very difficult situation. It's what our minds do. They are sense-making machines, if you will. Most of the time it serves us very, very well to have our minds making sense of our lives and the world. However, sometimes, especially when we are in a great deal of distress, our minds jump to worst case and very painful conclusions. My mind does the same thing. I think all minds can do that when under stress. It's sometimes worth slowing down the wheels a bit and considering whether the mind is jumping to some painful conclusions. If they are warranted, after all, we can still try to find ways to deal with tough situations. It's also important to know when we've made a jump that's not warranted by the facts.

ACT-Derived Strategies for Dealing with Painful Beliefs

A different set of cognitive interventions has arisen within what Hayes describes as Third Wave CBT (Hayes, 2004). Those are characterized by a greater emphasis on acceptance and mindfulness as well as strategies for working with the function of cognition, more than the form and frequency of cognition. In these therapies, little or no effort is put into trying to purposefully create alternative beliefs with the patient. Instead, experiences are created, often through metaphors and experiential exercises, during which the patient accesses a new place to stand in relation to a belief. The struggle with thoughts is dropped and inner experience is allowed to be present, but from a place which Hayes refers to as defusion. This is isomorphic to MBCT's emphasis on seeing thoughts as thoughts, rather than as facts, and metaphorically stepping back from them to watch them as though from a distance. For very entrenched beliefs, some of which have burdened the patient for many years, such techniques may offer an alternative set of strategies from those employed in traditional CBT. They provide the added benefit of insuring that the therapist refrains from engaging in a tug of war with the patient about what is true or correct to believe. As with any technique, done badly, the patient can feel dismissed and poorly understood, and the techniques can feel glib. But every intervention has its pitfalls, and the key is to use one well, see how it is received, rectify any breaches in the therapy relationship, and adjust accordingly (Safran & Segal, 1990).

As described in Chapter 2, humans process information at multiple levels, or in multiple modes. Experiential exercises, such as those developed in ACT, can speak, sometimes rapidly, to the more emotionally encoded information processing modes, sometimes with powerful and compelling results, while gently impacting the more explicitly verbal modes of information processing. In this sense, such interventions may operate in much the way that poetry does; by using emotionally laden imagery, an emotional impact can occur before the rational mind can grasp the meaning in words. In therapy, we want to help create experiences that can simultaneously target multiple levels of information processing, implicit and explicit, the more emotionally encoded meaning, and the more purely verbal level of meaning. In time, as one becomes familiar with the models, one can make up metaphors and exercises on the spot, with perhaps some of the most powerful interventions being derived from the metaphors that spontaneously appear in the patient's own language (Stott et al., 2010; Villatte et al., 2016).

Here's a technique that came from such a patient encounter, with Sally Klipsten, the depressed cancer patient whom we discussed earlier. The technique doesn't focus on changing the thoughts per se; it seeks to alter the controlling function of the thought by giving it a new function and meaning. It's called *There's a Parrot on My Shoulder.*

> Sally Klipsten and her husband owned pet birds, including a parrot, named Red. The therapist asked Sally to imagine that Red was on her shoulder and, using a light touch, asked Sally to "hear" Red saying some of the harsh things to Sally that Sally's own mind was saying, but in Red's parrot chattering voice. "It sounds silly when I hear Red say it," she spontaneously said. Asking her to consider how seriously she might take Red's word for it, she smiled and said, "He's just a bird." Asked further, if she would allow Red to drive her to the store, to run her life, or to make medical decisions, she laughed and said, "He's just a bird." "Suppose," the therapist said, "just suppose that our minds make noise at times, like Red does. How seriously ought we to take some of that noise?" "Not very," she answered. A bolder intervention might have the therapist and/or Sally say the words aloud, in a parrot's voice, together.

Notice that any intervention of this sort runs the risk of the patient feeling mocked or invalidated. By using the skills described in Chapter 3, and staying close to the patient's experience, respectfully, bolder interventions of this sort are not only tolerated well, they can open a fresh range of cognition and affect in session that can make change both compelling and even fun at times. Humor and playfulness, done well, may be one of the most powerful forms of promoting what ACT calls defusion, or that CBT refers to as distancing and de-centering. In this case, no effort is made to reduce the form or frequency of the painful belief. Rather, shifting its sound and its location to an imaginary parrot alters the function of the thought, its experience, and its impact. ACT has created a treasure trove of imaginative techniques, often in the form of guided imagery or other active, experiential exercises, built on the disciplined use of metaphors (Hayes et al., 2012; Stoddard & Afari, 2014). Understanding the theory behind ACT, Relational Frame Theory (RFT), can provide a platform from which such interventions can be both understood, and spontaneously created in session (Villatte et al., 2016).

Breaking Up Rumination

Treatment of rumination involves addressing the *process* rumination, without becoming ensnared in its content. Perhaps the first step in effectively pulling the plug on rumination is to know it for what it is, to recognize when one is ruminating, and to understand that it is in itself toxic. It stokes suffering, endlessly searching for answers to questions that have no answers ("What on earth is wrong with me?"), comparing oneself to a more ideal life, dredging up painful memories, stoking shame and sadness, and fueling depressive appraisals of self, one's place in the world, and future. In addition, time spent in rumination is time not spent engaging effectively with the world. Rumination dampens, rather than improves, problem-solving strategies (Harvey et al., 2004). It is important to note here that by fostering disengagement from rumination, we are not encouraging patients to avoid truly emotionally salient experience. When grief and loss are prominent, we encourage appropriate emotional expression in session. When the patient is faced with problems to deal with that may not have an easy solution, we enter into problem-solving mode with him or her. The behavior of rumination is a process that actually blocks the experience and expression of grief, and blocks effective problem solving. It is, itself, an inadvertent form of avoidance.

The first step in helping the depressed cancer patient out of the rumination trap is to help him or her see it for what it actually is: a colossal waste of time and a trap into a cycle of despondency. Psychoeducation about the nature of rumination and its role in deepening depression can be woven into the Guided Discovery and Socratic Questioning process, as the patient elicits the data to show how the patient is trapped in a vicious cycle of rumination. In addition, handouts providing psychoeducation about rumination can be accessed from www.psychologytools.com.

One technique is the use of a spatial metaphor. Here is an example of how it might be used with Todd Colvin:

THERAPIST: (Has a piece of paper and a pencil) Todd, from what you and your wife are saying, you spend a lot of time sitting in that dark room, thinking, thinking, imagining doom, wondering what you did wrong, what's wrong with you, and isolating yourself.

TODD: That's about it. Hours go by.

TODD'S WIFE: *Days* go by, and he doesn't even talk to me. I don't know what our future holds, but I want you back while you're here Todd.

THERAPIST: (Takes paper and draws a big circle on it) Todd, during times when you are in those dark hours, or days, how much space on this pie chart does your worry and rumination take up?

TODD: (Runs fingers around the entire outer circle) All of it. Damn near all of it.

THERAPIST: Does cancer, even in the tough spot you are in, deserve to take up all this space?

TODD: No. But it's really hard to get out of it. I hear my wife, though. The more I'm lying in bed alone, the less I'm with her and the kids. I just don't know what to do about that, though.

This is a subtle cognitive intervention, one that links the process of rumination to its painful and unintended consequences. It can set the stage for achieving some distance and de-centering from depressive ideation and to reduce the space that cancer takes up in the patient's life. Notice, too, that we are here utilizing one among many possible spatial metaphors to describe complex cognitive and behavioral processes, in a way that can often be easily understood and accepted by people. Linking rumination to the losses it creates, too, can be helpful. For every hour spent ruminating, an hour is lost with those who Todd Colvin cherishes the most in life: his wife and his children. Our central concerns are to help people unplug from rumination, without deepening their struggle with it. In addition, we also want to help people tune in to not only the consequences of rumination but also the lost opportunities to spend time in valued activities that is part of the cost of rumination. In turn, as we will see in a subsequent section, we help build behavioral repertoires and self-states that compete with and supplant states of extended rumination (Brewin, 2006; Bennett-Levy et al., 2015).

Just learning the function and cost of rumination may be enough for some cancer patients to pull their awareness, and their behavior, into other, more freely chosen, activities. However, many ruminators report feeling stuck and unable to discontinue rumination. Interventions targeting metacognitive beliefs may be indicated, with metacognitive beliefs including essentially beliefs about the mental operating system, or the workings of the mind. For example, continued rumination may be supported by what Wells called Type II metacognitive beliefs (Wells, 2000; 2009). Type II metacognitive beliefs include the belief that rumination is itself helpful, important, or necessary ("Rumination is helping me make sense of why I am such a loser") or, alternatively, the metacognitive belief that rumination is dangerous and that it signifies a mind that is dangerously out of control ("If I keep ruminating, I'll go crazy, or I'll make my cancer worse"). Wells (2000; 2009) described the kinds of cognitive processes that create these traps, including the belief that rumination serves a useful purpose or the belief that it is dangerous and out of control. A variety of attention training methods can be brought to bear on helping ruminators shift awareness from the inner stream of pain to five-senses experiences. For example, Wells used Attention Training techniques to help people tune in to sounds in the room, which appears to provide a rapid method of disengagement from internal processes (Wills & Sanders, 2013). Using brief periods of training, Wells has shown that these simple exercises, when presented cogently to the patient, and practiced briefly between sessions, can contribute to the patient's ability to shift awareness more freely to non-ruminative processes, which in turn can facilitate engagement in meaningful activity. With patients facing end-of-life concerns, or at least limitations in time, such interventions can help free them to more meaningfully engage with those they love, and in those activities that bring richness to life.

Sonja Lyubomirsky, a research psychologist who studies human happiness, wrote that when faced with illness, we can spend our time focusing on what the illness has taken away or cost us, on how it has ruined our lives. Or, we can focus on the people and activities that really matter to us. Quoting the psychologist and philosopher William James, she wrote, "One of my favorite quotes of all time is from William James: 'My experience is what I agree to attend to'" (Lyubomirsky,

2013, p. 187). While not all of our cancer patients can so freely shift attention to what matters, the anti-rumination techniques of CBT can help them do so.

Mindfulness in Treatment of Depression

Efforts to integrate mindfulness and self-processes into individual therapy are a work in progress. Segal et al. (2013) employed the "3-minute breathing space" in MBCT, which can be adapted for use in individual therapy in a way that allows for moments of grounding and safety as well as for introducing exposure to more emotionally charged and evocative experience. Metacognitive Therapy (MCT) utilizes its own version of mindfulness practice, called detached mindfulness, as well as attention training. The latter can be used to good effect in helping people gently train themselves to focus on external stimuli and cues, rather than remaining locked into ruminative processes (Wells, 2009; Wells & Fisher, 2016b). These techniques have the advantage of relative brevity as well as an empirical base to support their efficacy. Therapists at can access clinical and scientific material about MCT at www.mct-institute.com/metacognitive-therapy.

Let's turn to a clinical example of how we might implement a mindfulness intervention to help dampen the impact of rumination, by returning to the case of Todd Colvin. Once Todd was able to recognize the damaging effects of rumination and expressed a willingness to come back to the world, the following exercise could be tried:

THERAPIST: Todd, perhaps all of us could try an exercise together, if you're willing. (Todd and his wife agree) It's just a fairly simple exercise that won't ask a lot and that I'll do with you. It'll involve my asking you to sit up in a comfortable and straight posture. Just comfortably, spine comfortably straight, in a way that just supports our ability to breathe fully, from the belly to higher up in the lungs. If we sit hunched over, it sometimes compresses our ability to draw a breath. So notice when you get to a position of being straightened up, so the breath can be allowed in deeply. Nothing special here. Our bodies know when we arrive at that posture. Just a sense of dignity in the posture, maybe even a willingness to smile gently as you get into a position that's comfortable and dignified. And allowing in the breath, allowing the belly to fill as the air enters. If you'd like, you can take a moment to watch my hand, as I do this, myself. Then, allowing the breath to gently lift the diaphragm and rise. No need to hold the breath or force; just allow the body to breathe in as it knows how to do on its own.

The therapist then asks the patient to notice sounds in the room and to gently notice when the mind shifts to internal processes, such as thoughts, body sensations, memories, images, or emotions. When this inward focus asserts itself, the patient is encouraged to gently shift awareness to the posture and the breath, without struggle, without getting caught in judgments, and without expecting or insisting that one feel relaxed or happy. Just noticing. Not acting on anything that arises into awareness. Just cultivating the muscle of metacognitive awareness. Just practicing entering into a self-state of the observer. The therapist shifts from awareness of sounds in the room and outside the room to sensations in the body: pain, fatigue, whatever sensations arise. We then shift to emotions, then thoughts, always gently learning to bring awareness back to the breath, anchoring awareness in breath and posture, allowing thoughts, images, and emotions to just be present.

Even 5 to 10 minutes of this is often sufficient to produce the ability to push the pause button on suffering. Debriefing involves both asking the patient what he or she noticed and seeking to provide some discrimination training, between states of being caught in rumination versus a state of pause.

TODD: I noticed I felt sort of just here. Just being here in the room for a few minutes. I kind of liked it. I mean, I knew I still have a bad cancer. And all the stuff on my mind keeps coming in. But it was like I could just pause, like you said, and just be here.

TODD'S WIFE: Yeah. Me, too. It was really relaxing.

THERAPIST: Awareness can sometimes bring relaxation, sometimes not. Todd, could you give me a little more about what was happening when you were, as you said, just here?

TODD: Yeah. I just felt like, "Here I am. I'm not going anywhere right now. I don't have to be anywhere right now. I'm not dying right now. I'm not getting any surgery right now. I'm like, just here." And I liked that. Feels like I haven't been here in a while.

THERAPIST: In those moments, Todd, how much room was the cancer taking up?

TODD: In those moments? I guess it wasn't that much. Those moments didn't last very long, but no, in those moments that I was just here, no cancer was present.

Interventions of this sort need to be done, like any intervention, with considerable tact and with an eye toward the patient's capacity to engage. The objective is not to produce some dramatic epiphany or even to suggest that durable change occurs as a result of such a brief intervention. We are not trying to produce relaxation, though patients may well report a sense of ease during moments of pausing. Nor are we trying to chase away painful emotional states, as if sadness or fears were the enemy. In fact, we live in a culture in which painful emotions are easily conceived as the enemy, to be vanquished or obliterated. Mindfulness can be seen by many as one more strategy to keep painful feelings at bay. We are simply trying to open the door for the patient to fully enter the present moment in an open and accepting manner, one in which the non-cancer elements of the moment become accessible. The previous case vignette also demonstrates the way in which a variety of strands within CBT are woven together to help access, build, and anchor the patient in a self-state that fosters observing self in action and engaging with life. This included breath, posture, guided imagery, attention training, and metaphor, and draws on the science and theory outlined by Bennett-Levy et al. (2015), Korrelboom et al. (2012), and Brewin (2006). In addition, anchoring self in the present moment, with awareness of the non-cancer elements of the present moment, can also help access self-soothing states, and potentially downregulate an ongoing state of intense distress arousal (Gilbert, 2009a), with its attendant negative impact on emotional and physical health (Nezu et al., 2005; Lutgendorf & Anderson, 2015).

In delivering such interventions, we stay with the patient to monitor how an intervention is being experienced. If an intervention fails, we look for how or if this may have led to a possible breach in the therapy relationship, and we seek to rectify the relationship before proceeding (Safran & Segal, 1990). What we strive for is a moment in which the patient achieves even fleeting metacognitive awareness, optimally from the place of a dignified observing self.

Working with Self-Processes in Treating Depression

If depression fosters a sense of self as trapped, defeated, and hopelessness, one clinical strategy that has merit is working to foster self-states of strength and dignity. We might begin this process by fostering self-as-observer, derived from ACT, and consisting of briefly walking experientially with the person through various phases of his or her life, in which an observing self was always present, and remains so in this moment (Hayes et al., 2012). By fostering a more compassionate observing presence, self-processes conducive to facing and working with challenges, including cancer, can be built. Initial steps in this process involve fostering present moment awareness, through mindfulness exercises, as we have reviewed elsewhere. Exercises of this sort are always introduced and described, and permission is asked before proceeding. The therapist is wise to always make sure the patient is willing to give an exercise a try before launching into an experiential process that can be emotionally evocative. The therapist remains sensitive at all times to the patient's response during the exercise, as with mindfulness exercises, and titrates exposure to such experiential work according to patient response. This is followed by a guided imagery exercise, and before embarking on guided imagery, it is worth exploring with the patient how and even if he or she processes imagery (Hackmann et al., 2011). The process involves the following:

1. Noticing a self, observing and aware in the present moment;
2. Noticing that this observing self has been present in all experiences over the course of one's lifetime;
3. Inviting the patient to recall experiences as a child, combining pleasant and challenging experiences, in which an observing self was present;
4. Accessing memories from several points at later times in the patient's life, noticing the presence of an observing self, which runs like a continuous thread through the course of a life;
5. Bringing awareness of the observing self into the room again.

This can set the stage for another metaphor, also implemented via guided imagery, involving self as a bowl or container, capable of holding gently all experiences, painful, challenging, and joyous, with an untouched equanimity. Here is a highly condensed sample script, which can be added to the previous exercise:

> Now, allowing yourself to bring awareness to the present moment, with all the experiences of a lifetime resting here . . . just allowing life as it is to come to rest here, now, in this moment . . . the body sensations . . . the emotions . . . the thoughts . . . just as they are . . . bringing a gentle curiosity and a gentle caring to the noticing . . . with perhaps an awareness that this can all be here, held gently . . . as though this observing self is a lovely bowl, in which all experience can be held, allowed room . . . with room for it all . . . the body sensations . . . the emotions . . . memories . . . thoughts . . . just as they are . . . making room for life as it is.

This exercise can be implemented along with postures that support accessing compassionate, open, and observing self-processes: (Linehan, 2015) described "half smile and willing hands," for example, which adapts Buddhist practices for use with Western psychotherapy. Korrelboom et al. (2012; 2013) and Bennett-Levy et al. (2015) adapted the use of posture as a means of accessing and sustaining such changes. This exercise involves acceptance, metacognitive awareness, and the accessing of self-processes. These processes provide an alternative, to compete in memory retrieval (Brewin, 2006) with states of defeat and hopelessness. As in a classic ACT metaphor, The Chessboard Metaphor (Hayes et al., 2012), this is not about fostering a mental fight with oneself, as though two selves are fighting for access to awareness. Wilson et al. (2012) noted that self, from a behavioral perspective, is not a noun but a verb, a set of behavioral repertoires. Brewin's (2006) memory retrieval account suggested that we can build these processes in a manner that allows flexible and adaptive self-processes to emerge in place of the more dysfunctional processes into which one is pulled by depression.

ACT promulgates the idea that control is the problem, whereas Metacognitive Therapy (Wells, 2009) and MBCT are more inclined toward the idea that the *wrong* kind of control is the problem. For our purposes, we want to remain careful about the function served for the patient by our exercises. Rather than stoking avoidance of pain, our efforts involve the cultivation of a more compassionate and flexible ability to choose and alternate modes of being (Teasdale, 1999; Segal et al., 2013). Being with pain, even for a moment, in an open and spacious manner, with curiosity, gentleness, and compassion, can provide a glimpse of a new path to the waterfall. For patients who are interested, able, and willing, entry into ongoing MBSR or mindfulness programs for cancer patients may be indicated.

For another application of perspective-taking and self-processes with depressed cancer patients, let's turn to another case.

Carolyn Woods is a 46-year-old married mother of four, recovering from surgery, chemotherapy, and radiation for breast cancer. She had surgery 6 months ago and just completed a course of chemotherapy and radiation therapy. She has been told that she has good long-term recovery prospects and is now in the early stages of re-entry into survivorship. She has a history of prior depression and fears lapsing into what she calls "the darkness" she once experienced after the birth of her first child. She is currently mildly depressed and recognizes that she is not experiencing depression at the level she once did. In session she reveals not only mild depression and a fear of depression recurrence but also non-acceptance of the limitations imposed by her substantial surgical, chemotherapy, and radiation therapies. She is fatigued and she is distressed by changes in her physical appearance. However, what keeps coming to light in session is her sense that "I should be feeling better by now," "I can't afford to be tired like this," "I'm not being a good mother right now," and "What if I'm like this for the rest of my life?" This gap between how she is living and how imagines her life "should" be after treatment completion is fueling depression and suffering (Williams, M. et al., 2015).

Cognitive interventions of the sort outlined earlier could be effective. However, Carolyn indicates that many people have been telling her to "just be patient," which only irritates her. The therapist chose an experiential exercise that might not only bear fruit more rapidly but also could potentially bypass any strong reaction by the patient about being led forcefully toward acceptance and cognitive change by the therapist. The therapist asked Carolyn, along with her husband, Jack, who was in session, if they would be willing to do an exercise together with the therapist. The exercise would involve only some guided imagery, which they readily agreed to. Steve Hayes, a co-founder of ACT, created this exercise (Hayes, 2016). It involves asking the patient(s) to close eyes, sit as was described in the previous exercise with Todd Colvin, and make contact with whatever one is struggling with. In this case, Carolyn's struggle was with accepting the limitations she has in her life, following her cancer therapy: limited energy, heightened fatigue, and self-punishing beliefs. These can be seen as part of a vicious cycle of depression, with the cancer and the effects of treatment serving as activating events in the cycle. The exercise can be described in a sample transcript:

> Now noticing this struggle, allow yourself, if you will, to notice that you are noticing. It's as though there is a "you" inside your skin that is watching and observing this struggle. And if we walked through the course of a human life together, that you has most likely been there from the start of your having consciousness and is here today, now, in this body. Let yourself step out of this body, just for a moment, to look back on yourself, noticing the person you were 6 months ago, when you were told about the cancer. What do you think or feel about that person now, looking back? You don't have to answer this; but keep this in your awareness for now.
>
> Now, let's just sit here with the struggle you brought today. And as you look at this struggle, imagine that three years have gone by, and now you are looking back from a place of knowing how this will play out. (Pause) You are wiser, and looking back at yourself as you struggle today, imagine a message

you might want to pass across time to yourself now, from that wiser future self. Let's take a few moments to just be with this, seeing what message might come up, what advice you might give.

Let yourself, in your mind's eye, write down that message, allowing yourself to see it as though it were written on a piece of paper . . . now bring your awareness back to this room, here, now, and let's see if you can pass the message along, and if there is something in this message that might be useful for today's struggle.

Carolyn and her husband each received messages from a wise, future self. Carolyn's was simply: "Use your strength to accept how things have to be for now. In three years, you'll be better, and you'll be with Jack and the kids as the kids grow up." This message of acceptance and hope was literally self-generated and drew its power without any push or pull interaction with the therapist. While cognitive interventions may well have led to the same place, exercises of this sort can sometimes create change at multiple levels of information processing, and in a way that feels experientially compelling to the person. In this case, giving up the struggle with her body, tired, cut open, radiated, in pain and fatigued, helped create a more accepting posture toward re-entry into Carolyn's life.

Action Strategies: Linking Behavior to the Context of Daily Life

CBT's earliest roots lie in behaviorism. A contextually informed CBT helps the depressed cancer patient engage through behavior, not just through changing one's thoughts or appraisals. Two empirically supported therapies form a bedrock for action strategies in working with depressed cancer patients: Behavioral Activation and Problem-Solving Therapy.

Behavioral Activation with Cancer Patients

Evidence-based interventions, such as Behavioral Activation (BA) and Problem-Solving Therapies can be employed with depression at all levels of severity; however, these can be delivered in sometimes very brief therapy, including when depression severity in cancer patients is sub-syndromal, when distress seems linked to specific problems in the patient's daily life, and when it appears likely that the patient's distress will resolve or reduce when the key problems are effectively addressed (Mynors-Wallis & Lau, 2010). Many cancer patients do not present with substantial cognitive biases, and may thus be even more amenable to quick relief from depression, especially mild to moderate depression. Beck's CBT utilizes Activity Scheduling, particularly for the more severe depressions (A. Beck & Rush, 1979). Beckian activity scheduling is customarily designed to test depressive appraisals. BA evolved from a more behavioral tradition within psychology and generally eschews addressing the content of cognition in favor of its functions. Given the frequent absence of cognitive distortions in cancer patients, BA is perhaps more parsimonious and targeted to patient needs in many cases.

BA tunes in to two key behavioral and cognitive pathways into depression: avoidance of pain and loss of access to positively reinforcing experiences. One pathway into depression for cancer patients is the disruption in daily activities that cancer and its treatment can cause. Sometimes, brief, focused BA can help cancer patients reinstitute routines in a way that sparks a virtuous cycle. If pain, fatigue, recovery from treatment, and cognitive impairments are present, the therapist helps the patient scale his or her activities to what is possible, as a starting point, while also fostering acceptance of limitations. Richards (2010) described how BA can be employed as a low intensity intervention, delivered by less intensively trained CBT therapists. BA is a treatment that systematically helps people engage, or re-engage, in specific activities that are either pleasurable, necessary, or are routine daily behaviors, which have been disrupted by depression. Hopko adapted BA for briefer work, including for cancer patients (Hopko et al., 2003; Hopko et al., 2008).

Steps to implementing a BA plan are as follows:

1. Provide a rationale for how depression is related to the loss or disruption in daily routines, and the relationship between avoidance and depression;
2. Assess daily activities that have the potential to bring pleasure, that are necessary, and/or that are meaningful;
3. Create a hierarchy of activities, from those that are potentially most likely to be engaged in, to the most challenging;
4. Select behaviors to be engaged in between sessions, assuring reasonable likelihood of completion;
5. Use an activity scheduling form (www.psychologytools.com) to specify time, day, and activity to be carried out;
6. Identify and address potential barriers to completion, including cognitions, physical and energy limitations, impact of cancer and treatment, and so forth;
7. Review with the patient the potential beneficial impact of engagement in activity;
8. Review in next session;
9. Build new behavioral engagement strategies in follow-up session(s);
10. It can be useful to test predictions retrospectively, to see if the difficulties the patient anticipated in carrying out the activities matched their experience, making this akin to a behavioral experiment (Bennett-Levy et al., 2004).

Case Example

June is a 56-year old woman, living with bone pain, at times quite acute, from multiple myeloma. She is divorced and lives with a son, who is 19 and working full time. She has had the disease for nearly 5 years and is now on disability. Due to recent fractures and attendant pain, she has withdrawn from friends, from taking walks, and from leaving home. She has become increasingly irritated, which she fears has, in turn, alienated her son. Depression was revealed to be mild to moderate in severity. June presents with many adaptive strengths, including a sense of humor, and considerable resourcefulness, acceptance, and wisdom in dealing with cancer. Her most acute pain has subsided, through the healing of a recent rib fracture as well as pain medications provided by the palliative care team. However, her mood remains low, and engagement in pleasurable and necessary daily activities has declined. June is receiving chemotherapy, and her daily life is organized around her chemo schedule, including recovery time between visits to the hospital. A rationale was provided, regarding the link between mood and activities as well as how cancer's contributions to a restricted life can contribute to depression. A focus on reclaiming her life from cancer followed, including identifying behaviors that could bring pleasure, others that were necessary for daily life (re-establishing grooming and hygiene routines, exercise, diet), and those that would be meaningful (restoration of her relationship with her son). June chose the following:

1. Contact one close friend, with whom she had not spoken in weeks;
2. Set alarm clock for 7:00 a.m., and then follow a schedule including coffee, toast, showering, and dressing;
3. Take a 10-minute walk daily, now that pain has subsided;
4. Speak with her son about her irritability from the bone pain and seek to restore their relationship.

Implementation barriers were identified and addressed. In the following chemotherapy visit, a week later, June had her activity schedule, showing that she had called and set up a coffee date with her friend and that she had walked twice for 10 minutes. And she was able to have a productive talk with her son, in which he revealed that when she was in such pain, he feared losing her to cancer. June's mood was improved from this intervention.

Infusing BA with Meaning and Values

Motivation and willingness to engage in both BA and problem-solving approaches can be strengthened by linking them to the patient's values and to the sources of meaning in their lives. Values and meaning form the bedrock of Victor Frankl's (1986; 1992) work and Irvin Yalom's (1980) work, and they inform other approaches to working with end-of-life issues with cancer patients (Breitbart et al., 2010; Breitbart & Poppito, 2014). Within the CBT tradition, particularly as introduced through ACT, values can serve as verbally constructed motivators, intrinsic sources of meaning, and guides to action (Dahl et al., 2009; Hayes, Villatte et al., 2011; Villatte et al., 2016). In turn, value-guided actions help create a self-sustaining virtuous cycle.

There are ample resources to help therapists to assess values and areas of meaning in life (Dahl et al., 2009; Wilson et al., 2010). An example of a worksheet that can be used to help patients make contact with important values can be found on www.psychologytools.com. This ACT worksheet can also be used to help vitalize and set a course for therapy, is public domain, and is adapted from Wilson et al. (2010). Important life values often include areas such as "being with and there for my family," "being a friend," "being there for others as a citizen and neighbor," and "helping others." Other life domains include spiritual development, health behaviors, recreational activities, work activities, and service to others. It is important to note that a value is not the same as a goal. Goals may have end points: "I want to get rich enough to retire early." Values never end, and a single step in the direction of a value is itself living the value. It is an ongoing process, to be nurtured, and to be re-engaged whenever we realize we have moved away from that, by avoidance, or by engagement in an action that pulls us away from what truly matters.

Linking patient strengths and values to action involves finding ways in which a value shows up in the seemingly small steps that are achievable, given any limitations imposed by cancer. Villatte et al. (2016) provided clinical applications of Relational Frame Theory (RFT), including what they refer to as hierarchical framing, which have utility in working with cancer patients. In particular, cancer patients who have lost areas of functioning, due to the cancer and its treatment, may benefit from interventions that target possible meaningful actions, even within the limits imposed by cancer and its treatments. Experiential exercises, involving perspective taking and hierarchical framing, can help the person link values to specific behaviors consistent with those values, and can foster behavioral engagement. Steps to do this are as follows:

1. Connect to self-experience;
2. Contact values;
3. Describe actions that are consistent with those values;
4. Describe valued actions that are possible given infinite time, money, and resources;
5. Scale back time, money, and resources, finding ways that one's values can show up with just this moment, just this place, with no money, and no other resources;
6. Identify specific behaviors possible now, in this moment.

Even without a detailed knowledge of RFT, ACT techniques can be powerful and can be utilized to good effect by competent CBT therapists (Villatte et al., 2016). Matthieu Villatte, PhD, offers training in RFT, including clinical applications relevant to cancer work, at The Practice Ground: www.practiceground.org.

For a patient like Sally Klipsten, who values being a loving grandmother, her limitations in energy and time have led her to conclude that she cannot be a loving grandmother unless she is her old self. She then discounts the many steps that she still takes, and can yet take, to be a loving grandmother, even if there is little time, less energy, increased pain. Here is a sample of a clinical dialogue, targeting these processes experientially:

THERAPIST: So you're saying that you can't be the grandmother you want to be, now that you have this diagnosis?

SALLY: I won't be there for graduations or weddings, and the little ones won't even remember me when they get older.

THERAPIST: So being remembered is important, right?

SALLY: Yes, and just missing out on being with them all. Our family gets together at holidays. When all the kids are in town, we sometimes go to Mass together on Christmas or Easter. We celebrate birthdays. And I was hoping to retire soon and go to sports events and other activities with the grandkids. Now I won't be able to do those things, and they won't remember me. Plus, I'm so tired right now that I can't even do the things that I want to do while I'm alive.

THERAPIST: How are memories formed of people?

SALLY: Well, I guess by being together. And I suppose by things like photographs or videos, I guess.

THERAPIST: OK. Yeah, I think those are good ways to describe how we form memories of people who are important in our lives. Would you be willing to do a brief imagery exercise with me, just a little guided imagery exercise that we can do together, all of us? (Sally's husband is in the consultation room as well)

SALLY: I guess so. Sure. (Husband agrees also)

THERAPIST: (Introduces mindfulness as in prior experiential examples, settling into chairs, sitting in a dignified posture, focus on breathing and noticing self experiences. Then invites patient and her husband to open eyes and bring attention and awareness back to the room). OK, you said that building memories and being with your kids and grandkids is important to you. What is it about that that is important to you?

SALLY: Well, just loving them, I guess, and just their knowing that grandma loves them and is with them.

THERAPIST: If you had all the time in the world, and all the money in the world, how would you show them you love them and are with them? What actions would you do?

SALLY: Oh my. I'd go to all their games, all their life cycle events forever. I'd hug them and kiss them, and I'd tell them all, my kids and my grandkids that Grandma believes in them. (Tears form in her eyes) I'd have them over for dinner pretty often, and I'd cook, which I can't really do now like I used to. And we'd pay for all their college educations (Laughs and looks at husband, who nods)

HUSBAND: But we don't have that kind of money.

THERAPIST: Yeah, sure, but we're talking about if there was endless time and endless money, right? So OK, now let's say that you have 6 months, and

I'm not saying that's what you have. I don't know. Nobody knows. But let's just say this as a thought. Six months. No more money than you have. What would you do to be the loving mom and grandma that matters to you?

SALLY: Well, I guess I couldn't pay for their college. And I don't have the energy to get to all their games. And I can't cook dinners for everyone.

THERAPIST: Well, let's say a small step, if you were just sitting here in the chair, and a grandchild was in the room. What could you do to show loving grandma?

SALLY: I could say, "I love you," "I believe in you." I could give them a hug and a kiss.

THERAPIST: I see. And how are memories formed?

SALLY: Well, I guess by hugs, kisses, "I love yous," and "I believe in yous." And if I can't cook dinner, I can make some cookies and have them over.

THERAPIST: So is being a loving grandmother something that can happen now, even as things are?

SALLY: Yes.

Therapy involved helping Sally set about creating good times and potentially enduring memories with her children and, especially, her grandchildren. A grand-mother-grandchildren sleepover, with videos and photos, as well as other legacy projects, provided realistic comfort that her impact on her progeny would be enduring. And in the meantime, more vitality was to be extracted from life, even though it would remain tinged with sadness and impending grief.

Elvira, whose case formulation we reviewed in the last chapter, was constrained by not only her illness but also by financial and marital limitations. In addition, long-standing beliefs in her subjugation and in the importance of avoiding con-flict created limitations in accessing a greater and more flexible range of behav-ioral and problem-solving options. The therapist sensed that these limitations were not flexible, either on Elvira's part or within her marital relationship. Given that our therapy is of necessity often brief and is focused on the resolution or the management of current challenges, we may be obliged to work within the limita-tions of the personal and social context(s) in which they are embedded. This, too, requires flexibility, inventiveness, and acceptance by the therapist. Setting the main problem as that of establishing more frequent personal contact with her daughter and grandchildren, the therapist worked with Elvira to make this happen. Elvira began by learning how to use FaceTime on her iPhone scheduling regular talk time with her daughter and grandchildren. She and her daughter found ways to pay for travel together, and Elvira booked a five-day visit, which would turn into a reunion with other family members who would join for part of the time. Her husband remained at home, and she acknowledged that he would likely remain detached and distant.

ACT teaches that one's most cherished values have as their flip side pain: an ACT saying goes, "In your values are your pain, and in your pain are your values." For Todd Colvin, turning from the wall and re-engaging with his wife and children was fraught with pain. He would not be able to look at his wife without knowing that his time with her was likely to be very limited. In the midst of contact with his children, he would have moments of deep sadness and grief, tinged with fear, at the knowledge that he would not likely be there to protect and guide them on their life journeys. Todd's many strengths included his fierce loyalty and love of his family, his work ethic, his sense of honor and integrity, his belief in the importance of friends, in civic service, and in his church. By engaging those strengths and committing to a value-driven course of action, he was free to problem solve, to create a legacy project, and to live as fully as possible in the time he had left. In Todd Colvin's case, this meant working directly with Todd and his wife, conjointly, to problem solve a course of action that would insure the family's financial survival in the likely event of his death from cancer. His wife chose to return to school, which she had left after the birth of their first child. Todd experienced relief, knowing that while he did not make a fortune to leave behind, he had married a woman who would find a path to survive and flourish. She would become an accountant. A video he made, with his thoughts and wishes for his oldest son, would be there, with his son, on his son's high school graduation day, in two years. In the meantime, there were bike rides, a trip for a family reunion, and the small pleasures of which daily life can be composed. Depression did not go on the trips with Todd, just the painful, bittersweet sadness of his circumstances.

Problem-Solving Strategies

Strategies from Problem-Solving Therapy (PST) are especially suited to patients whose depression is associated with everyday problems and whose depression may be less entrenched in rumination and withdrawal. Many cancer patients present with sub-syndromal depression, and the added distress of the daily difficulties associated with managing cancer is a contributing factor to depression, making PST techniques highly relevant to our treatment efforts. To return to our earlier use of the juggler metaphor, we can set the stage to normalize problems in life and to engage the patient in a renewed problem-solving effort. PST is a manualized therapy, whose format is readily adopted for work with cancer patients.

Problem-solving therapies (PST) formed an early part of the development of Cognitive Behavior Therapy (Spivack et al., 1976) and have evolved into efficacious treatments for depression, and health problems, including cancer, (Schwartz et al., 1998; Nezu et al., 1999; Perri et al., 2001; Nezu et al., 2005;). PST also forms a core of skills used in DBT, as Interpersonal Effectiveness skills. The United Kingdom's IAPT (Improving Access to Psychological Therapies) program included problem-solving therapy as a low-intensity treatment for depression, making it suitable as a therapy for which non-doctoral personnel might be trained to deliver it. The UK's National Institute for Clinical Excellence (NICE) Clinical Practice Guidelines for Depression (2009) included PST "as an appropriate intervention for patients with mild to moderate depressive disorder" (Mynors-Wallis & Lau, 2010, p. 151).

PST techniques fit directly into our case formulation model by assessing and defining specific problems to be included in a problem list. In cases where the person is overwhelmed from juggling, or where the person's view of self leads to avoidant or ineffective problem-solving strategies, PST can provide a simple set of strategies to implement in possibly few sessions. It also dovetails with all our efforts to help people find another way of viewing self and circumstances, one that lends itself to problem solution, problem acceptance, and reduced suffering in the face of life challenges. The use of the juggler metaphor (Chapter 2) can be used to explain how our problem-solving efforts can be swamped when we face juggling more items in our life than our emotional and cognitive resources allow for. In turn, PST techniques can help reinstate a sense of self as capable, engaged, and effective.

A clear, brief description of PST is available in Mynors-Wallis and Lau (2010). Clear problem definitions are achieved, and links between patient distress and the problems are shown. Problems include situations that are causing suffering, and for which change strategies are warranted. Refusal to accept reality, such as "I just want this to go away," is not a viable target for a change strategy. Similarly, "I need for my doctor to be likable" is not a workable problem, since it is not directly in the control of the patient. "I want to find ways to cooperate and work effectively with my doctor, even though I don't like him or her very much" *is* a potentially workable problem definition. The patient and therapist then clearly focus on a key problem, with attention paid to when the problem occurs, where it occurs, and who is involved with the problem. Interpersonal issues are not uncommonly implicated in problems, and this can include communication difficulties with members of the oncology team, with family, co-workers and bosses, or with friends. Other problems can include working within the limitations imposed by cancer: how much exercise can be engaged in without increasing pain and fatigue, how to achieve and provide sexual satisfaction when sexual functioning is affected by cancer and therapy, how to cope with the uncertainty and waiting periods between follow-up visits with the oncology team.

Once problems are clearly specified, the patient and therapist begin generating a list of possible alternative problem-solving strategies, without initially worrying about which ones will work. After a list is developed, the therapist and patient generate a list of pros and cons for each possible solution, as they begin to evaluate each possible strategy to find one that seems most likely to address the problem. Planning then occurs to describe how to go about implementing this strategy, including anticipating potential barriers as well as thinking through ways to address possible barriers. Implementation of the problem-solving strategy is followed in a subsequent session by assessing whether the strategy achieved its intended effects. Modifications can be made as needed. A paradigm is created between the therapist and patient, in which problems in life are normalized and are viewed as challenges to be met with curiosity and ingenuity. A method is created for generating alternative problem-solving strategies, prioritizing them, implementing them, and testing them in terms of their outcome.

The Case of the Radioactive Woman

Sylvia Janes is a 32-year-old married woman who presents with a newly diagnosed ovarian cancer for which radiation therapy is the first treatment option. She and her husband, Hugh, have no children. A referral was made, due to concerns that she was depressed. The PHQ-9 revealed moderate depression, though of short duration, and in the interview Sylvia explained her concerns. She has been worried about the diagnosis she received, yet is confident in her medical team, including the treatment strategy that they selected. She has had six treatments and is scheduled for another 24. Her primary concern is that she feels isolated, including from her husband, who she said has been staying away from her, not touching her or comforting her as she is accustomed to him doing. She mentioned that he had been asking her if she would become dangerously radioactive once she started therapy. He appeared to be shying away from contact with her and recently began sleeping in another bedroom. She has told him that her radiation poses no danger to him, but he continues to distance himself. Sylvia is increasingly lonely, and although she has friends and other family support, she relies on Hugh, in what has otherwise been a close marriage.

Sylvia's depression was of recent onset, and a single episode. The loss of social support from her husband, and his difficulties touching, being near, or understanding her, seemed to be key activating events. She did not present with cognitive features of depression, in terms of significant cognitive biases or distortions. Her portrayal of her husband was that he was a loving yet simple man, who would not listen to her about the safety of the radiation therapy. Sylvia defined the problem as loss of her husband's understanding and his physical proximity. While one could conclude that this problem definition was not in her control, making an effort to reach her husband was something that she did want to pursue. The therapist explored the strategies that Sylvia had already used, to no avail. These included her telling him that she was not radioactive. We generated a list of potential alternative strategies to reach Hugh:

1. Ask him to talk with the radiation oncologist;
2. Find online resources, recommended by the oncology staff, for him to read;
3. Ask him to speak with another family member who had undergone radiation therapy.

In assessing the pros and cons of each alternative, Sylvia believed that the oncologist would be threatening to her husband. But she thought that if someone else on the team could speak with him, perhaps one not threatening to him, they might get through. The therapist and Sylvia named each person on the oncology team, and there was one particular nurse on the team who she thought might have the balance of kindness and a no-nonsense demeanor that might reach Hugh. The therapist invited the nurse into the session, and she readily agreed to meet with Hugh and Sylvia, along with the therapist. Sylvia role-played with the therapist how she would ask Hugh to talk about his concerns, knowing that he would be bringing her to the hospital later that week. In session with the nurse, Hugh brought up his concerns only after Sylvia spoke for him, with his permission, and as they had agreed to prior to the session. The nurse definitively reassured Hugh and Sylvia that she was not radioactive and that the best thing for them both, under the circumstances, was physical and emotional closeness, "the more the merrier." In follow-up consultation between the nurse and the therapist, Sylvia's mood had improved as her husband's physical and emotional support returned to normal.

A last case is in order, to demonstrate multiple components of intervention in dealing with cancer-related depression. This case also demonstrates how depression can appear as a first episode, even deep in long-term survivorship from cancer.

The Case of the Man Who Was Turning into Stone

Depression in survivorship can occur many years after successful intervention for cancer. Let's turn to the case of Richard Kelly, 57, who survived surgery for a nasopharyngeal cancer, and full-head radiation therapy, more than 20 years prior to his first behavioral health consultation. The impact of the surgery had been speech and language difficulties, associated with removal of part of the tongue, jaw, and palate. He had lost all his teeth, removed prior to embarking on full-head and neck radiation therapy. Yet he had not only survived, he had maintained a full-time career in a physically demanding profession. He had reared two sons into adulthood, re-married following a divorce when the children were young, and maintained a workout routine that was as demanding as his job, as a line supervisor in a refrigerator manufacturing plant. Now, more than 20 years later, the cumulative impact of treatment was taking a toll on his body and his mood. Full-head and neck radiation had produced neuropathy, which was causing painful muscle contractions and hardening of the muscle tissue. All areas that had received radiation were affected: head, neck, throat, and upper back. Over the past 2 to 3 years, Richard's muscles had become increasingly tight, hard, and knot-like. A massage therapist he had worked with said that she had never seen muscles that were so tight, hard, and unyielding. "I feel like my body is turning into stone," he said. Additionally, Richard was having more difficulty swallowing, because of the radiation therapy's long-term impact. He had recently begun to choke, even when eating small pieces of food. His diet was becoming increasingly restricted, cutting off one source of pleasure for him, and reducing him to soups and other liquids as well as eggs and other soft foods.

Pain had become so constant and unremitting, as had the muscle contractions, that he was exhausted by the end of the day, and retreated to his bedroom, depressed and irritable. He had recently taken leave, using the Family and Medical Leave Act (FMLA) for extended time away from work. The demands of his job—a source of pride, independence, money, meaning, and social contact—was now out of the picture. He was no longer able to maintain the fierce workout routine that he had proudly and rather defiantly maintained in the face of all the challenges that cancer had posed for him. He prided himself on maintaining a strong, muscular physique, even though the cancer had affected his face and his speech. Now, he said, looking into a mirror "I see a wrecked old man looking back at me." He was lacking in energy to spend as much quality time with his adult children and grand-children as he once had, provide care to his aging widowed father, or enjoy time with his wife. He maintained a strong will to live but was increasingly preoccupied by visual images of himself sitting in a wheelchair, choking, and eventually dying of the long-term effects of his treatment. Richard also was upset that he was not able to get clear answers about his medical status, and that there was disagreement between the pain team, the palliative care team, and his other medical providers about how best to manage pain and quality of life issues. Therapy focused on the following:

1. Acceptance work related to the losses he was accruing from his medical status.
2. Acceptance work also included dealing with the medical unknowns of his long survivorship and the fact that his medical team had not seen someone with his set of concerns so far out from the diagnosis and treatment of cancer. In this sense, the team worked to help slow the prospect of ending as he envisioned herself, in a wheelchair.
3. Problem solving with Richard to help him choose a strategy regarding pain management, which he elected to be managed by the palliative care team.
4. Helping Richard develop a life management plan that included massage therapy (with the blessings of the palliative care specialist), yoga, and mindfulness meditation.
5. In-session mindfulness exercises, including use of mindfulness of breath to create moments-to-pause.
6. Self-process work to help Richard access the wise and compassionate self that remained present in his deteriorating body.
7. Setting priorities regarding which life values mattered most. This set the stage for problem-solving strategies, which helped him decide to retire from his career and accept disability status. While this represented a loss of income, independence, social contact, and meaning, it also cre-ated more opportunities to conserve energy, protect himself from the abusive effects on his body of his job, and to spend quality time with his wife, children, grandchildren, and his aging father.

Chapter Summary

This chapter addressed the varied presentation of depression in cancer patients. This includes patients who meet criteria for *DSM* syndromal depression as well as the many patients who have sub-syndromal depression. Patient presentations that include depressive adaptation to the physical effects of cancer were addressed. The transdiagnostic model for formulating cancer-related depression led to a description of a full spectrum of interventions available to the clinician. These included dealing with depressive beliefs, helping patients access a more resilient sense of self, breaking up rumination, and fostering active engagement in meaningful and necessary activities of daily life.

Key Points

1. Cancer-related depression is more common than depression in the general population, though its features may differ in several ways: there may be fewer frank cognitive distortions; the sense of self as overwhelmed, helpless, and trapped may be prominent; sub-syndromal presentations related to adjustment difficulties may be frequent; cancer-related physical symptoms are often implicated in assessing and treating depression.

2. Rapid screening for depression is necessary and can include a general screener, such as the Edmonton Symptom Assessment System-Revised (ESAS-R) and the PHQ-9. These serve to help focus the clinical interview, where transdiagnostic features of depression can be targeted for inquiry and intervention.

3. A provisional hierarchy of intervention strategies for depressed cognitive content was provided.

4. Strategies for problematic cognitive content include a continuum of interventions, ranging from soft style Beckian probes, to Beckian restructuring techniques, to more experiential interventions intended to rapidly alter the patient's relationship to problematic content.

5. Rumination as a toxic process, cognitively and behaviorally, must be assessed and strategies implemented that help the patient identify rumination when it occurs, choose to shift awareness away from internal processes, and re-engage in necessary, pleasurable, and/or meaningful activities in the moment.

6. A focus on self-processes is important, to help patients access and strengthen the sense of self as capable of meeting the challenges posed by cancer, and to live meaningfully in the face of those challenges.

7. Mindfulness experiential exercises can be incorporated into individual and couple sessions, even when patients have not had prior experience in such programs as MBCT. These can include guided imagery exercises, and incorporation of five-senses activities, including breathing, for purposes of helping to push the pause button on suffering. This, in turn, can help access self-processes related to maintaining engagement and a fighting spirit.

8. Two low-intensity empirically supported interventions for depression in cancer patients can be implemented to restore daily routines (Behavioral Activation) and to promote effective problem-solving (Problem-Solving Therapy).

Seven
Treating Anxiety in Cancer Patients

Although nearly 65% of cancer patients will likely survive to 5 years after diagnosis (Stanton et al., 2015), each person who survives cancer nonetheless lives with the specter of recurrence and death. Cancer is rightly experienced as a potentially grave threat to one's life and to one's sense of self. In addition, the demands of treatment, and its effects, can also be experienced as highly stressful and fraught with potential threats, making cancer fertile soil for the blossoming of clinically significant anxiety. Anxiety is the most common psychological problem among those newly diagnosed with cancer and especially those who are experiencing a recurrence of disease. Combined with depression, perhaps a third of cancer patients (Moorey & Greer, 2012; Jacobsen & Andrykowski, 2015) may experience significant distress. Cancer-related worry can be ubiquitous, depending upon the nature of the diagnosis, the stage of treatment, and the cancer journey of the individual patient. As in depression, the clinician is called upon to treat both syndromal and sub-syndromal anxiety, with the latter, consisting primarily of adjustment problems, being the most common.

At heart, anxiety is rooted in fear states. And the capacity to experience fear is an evolutionarily adaptive response to threat. Beck's theory is connected to evolutionary psychology and biology in the sense that threat sensitivity confers enormous adaptive advantages by alerting, orienting, and preparing the organism to engage with threat via fight, flight, or freeze responses. Yet in contrast to fear, anxiety involves a more prolonged state of fear arousal (D.A. Clark & Beck, 2012) maintained by psychological and cognitive processes unique to humans. Both Beck and newer models of CBT recognized that one key difference between fear and anxiety rests in human language (Beck & Emery, 1985; Eifert & Forsyth,

2005; Villatte, Hayes et al., 2011; D.A. Clark & Beck, 2012). This unique human capacity for language allows us to anticipate and effectively plan for future threats and opportunities; yet it contains within itself a curse that is unique to humans (Hayes, Villatte et al., 2011; Kabat-Zinn, 2013). The ability to imagine a future, and the ability to experience fear arousal in response to one's imagined future, or to one's own thoughts, body sensations, and emotions, create conditions for humans to potentially enter a constant state of threat arousal. Animals turn off their fear systems when the threat has passed; humans can respond to psychological threats in a way that never allows the fear system to subside (Sapolsky, 2004).

For some patients, a diagnosis of cancer exacerbates a pre-existing state of chronic stress arousal, flooding the body with a cascade of stress hormones, affecting sleep, appetite, mood, concentration, and problem-solving abilities. In some cases, these processes can continue far into survivorship. For others, the episodes of stress arousal and anxiety are transient, such as in response to a diagnosis of cancer, or in response to facing surgical, radiation, or chemotherapies. Similarly, fear arousal can occur at intervals, such as when cued by return visits for monitoring their disease status, and while awaiting the results of scans and other tests. Medical phobias and symptoms of post-traumatic stress disorder are more likely among those who have endured cancer therapy than in a general population (Jacobsen & Andrykowski, 2015; Salmon et al., 2015). These anxiety problems, too, can affect adherence to treatment regimens, including engagement in monitoring and follow-up.

If, as a starting point, we focus on Beck's cognitive model for understanding anxiety disorders, we note that it rests on a seemingly simple heuristic: anxiety is a function of one's threat appraisals and one's beliefs about one's ability to manage threat. Beck's model led to the development of an "anxiety equation" (Salkovskis, 1996a; Butler et al., 2008; Wills & Sanders, 2013), which states:

$$\text{Anxiety} = \frac{\text{Perceived likelihood that threat will occur} \times \text{Perceived cost / awfulness}}{\text{Perceived ability to cope} + \text{Perceived rescue factors}}$$

The numerator in this equation, perceived threat × the perceived cost/awfulness, often contains misappraisals of threat, or overestimations of threat, in Beck's model. In cancer, while there may indeed be misappraisals and cognitive biases, the threat is often very, very real. Cancer can, and does, pose existential threats, and its treatments can be both awful and costly, even when the outcome is survival. So in cancer-related anxiety states, we might expect the numerator in the anxiety equation to be generally high and not necessarily fraught with overestimations of threat. Yet the same cognitive biases that characterize other anxiety disorders can occur in cancer patients: catastrophizing, jumping to conclusions, selective attention, nearsightedness, emotional reasoning, and all-or-none thinking (D.A. Clark & Beck, 2010; 2012).

In addition to possible misappraisals of threat, which show up in the *content* of thinking and imagery, a person can respond to cancer by engaging in a toxic *process*: runaway worry. To worry is human. To worry after receiving a diagnosis of cancer is nearly inevitable (Levin et al., 2010). Yet worry that takes certain forms, and becomes chronic, can stoke considerable suffering (Borkovec, 2006; Wells, 2009), including the potential for states of chronic stress arousal. Rumination and worry share many common properties, and both can be present in depression and anxiety disorders, as some of the case examples from the last chapter on depression demonstrated. For heuristic purposes, worry tends to be more centered on the future, while rumination often involves turning the mental lens on the past. Both the mental *content* of fear states, and the recursive *processes* of worry, can stoke psychophysiological suffering, impede effective problem solving and coping, and deepen a sense of isolation and helplessness. As noted earlier, there is now accumulating evidence that the forms of worry identified by Wells (2009) are associated with anxiety disorders and depression in cancer patients (Cook et al., 2015). Targeting those processes in CBT is, therefore, vital.

The science of psychology is increasingly contributing knowledge, embedded in the theories and techniques of modern CBT that can help people live once, more fully, as we will address in this chapter. As foundational as Beck's model has been in the treatment of cancer patients, newer models of CBT have added to our scientific, theoretical, and technical ability to treat anxiety problems (Eifert & Forsyth, 2005; Borkovec, 2006; Robichaud & Dugas, 2006; 2009; Forsyth & Eifert, 2008; Hayes, Villatte et al., 2011; Mansell et al., 2013). Our work with the numerator in the anxiety equation involves assessing and intervening in both cognitive content and cognitive processes, when they go awry. As part of our assessment of the patient's threat estimations, we may become involved in helping patients obtain information about their illness, their prognosis, and what their treatments entail. This, in turn, may involve interfacing with the treatment team on the patient's behalf, or by helping the patient deal more effectively with the team. When the patient's threat estimations are overblown, and when systematic cognitive biases are implicated in stoking anxious arousal and dampening effective engagement in treatment, we address those biases in cognitive content. We'll look at some examples of how to do this work in later sections of this chapter.

The denominator of the equation suggests that anxiety is also a function of one's perceived ability to cope, plus one's belief that rescue factors are available. Rescue factors, in the case of cancer, may involve the expectation of cure, or the prolongation of life. It may involve the sense that one is spiritually or religiously protected. It may involve the belief that medicine will be available to help manage pain and nausea, or trust in one's medical team, and the support of others, including partners, family members, friends, co-workers, and spiritual communities. Much of our effort in treating anxiety in cancer patients consists of helping patients increase their denominator. This involves employing the key principles we have developed in this book to do two things. First, we help increase the patient's ability to manage the threats and costs of cancer; second, we help to increase the social, medical, and other supports necessary to improve the patient's sense that he or she has allies in facing their struggle.

The key processes that maintain anxiety problems and foster and maintain vicious cycles of anxiety include the following:

1. Misappraisals of threat;
2. Intolerance of uncertainty;
3. Worry, including thoughts and imagery;
4. Selective attention for internal and external threat cues;
5. Limited capacity for present moment awareness;
6. Underestimation of personal resources for managing threat;
7. Experiential avoidance;
8. Limited distress tolerance abilities;
9. Ineffective problem-solving strategies.

We will address these factors when we focus on clinical strategies for managing anxiety in cancer patients. Those strategies use the principles outlined in Chapter 2, and involve the following:

1. Managing the therapeutic relationship with anxious cancer patients;
2. Incorporating psychoeducation into the treatment, to both normalize fear and set the stage for acceptance and/or change;
3. Dealing with threat appraisals, cognitive biases, uncertainty intolerance, and worry;
4. Entering the present moment via mindfulness and acceptance practices;
5. Building distress tolerance and emotion regulation skills;
6. Accessing and building resilient self-processes;
7. Connecting to meaning and purpose via active engagement in the face of threat and uncertainty.

Not all of the possible maintaining factors are necessarily present in each case. And not all of the clinical strategies are necessarily brought to bear on each case. The therapist selects treatment targets, relevant core processes, and interventions based on the formulation for any given patient.

Managing the Therapy Relationship with Anxious Patients

The use of screening instruments, including the ESAS-R and the Generalized Anxiety Disorder Scale (GAD-7), in addition to a handoff by other members of the treatment team, allows the therapist to home in on relevant patient concerns in the first session. One can further assess worry, as needed, by using the Penn State Worry Questionnaire (Meyer et al., 1990) or the Metacognitions Questionnaire 30 (MCQ-30) (Wells, 2009). Assessment of the patient also requires explaining to patients what treatment options are available, with what evidence base for each.

While the focus of this book is on psychotherapy, the use of medication to manage depression and anxiety is also routinely offered as an option. Patient preferences for one treatment over another, or in combination, should always be taken into account. Patients who are immediately facing highly distressing diagnoses and procedures, and for whom distress tolerance is limited, may benefit considerably from at least the short-term use of anxiolytics and/or SSRIs or other anti-depressant/anti-anxiety medications. Similarly, when significant sleep difficulties are intruding on adaptive functioning, medication on perhaps a short-term basis can be a value adjunct to treatment. It is advisable to work collaboratively with the oncology teams on questions of medication; many oncology teams have medical oncologists, psychiatrists, physician's assistants, or doctoral-level nurses who are comfortable prescribing anti-depressants and anti-anxiety medications.

With respect to clinical interviews, the same principles of Guided Discovery and Socratic Questioning are used in treating anxiety disorders as in depression. The presence of a caring therapist, who is not afraid to walk with the patient through the entire experience of their cancer, is vital. Simply having a place to talk openly about cancer can be both a relief for some patients and a form of exposure to fear-eliciting cues. At the same time, anxious patients may be prone to emotion dysregulation if GD/SQ is not done with considerable sensitivity and if the pace of the session is too brisk (Butler et al., 2008). Although experiential avoidance needs to be spotted in working with cancer patients, we are more likely to see patients who are immersed in fear states. In contrast to clinical presentations of anxiety in non-cancer patients, cancer patients are often already immersed in fear-generating situations on a daily basis, having been thrown into the deep end of the sea, first by a diagnosis of cancer, then by the demands and effects of treatment. Preserving a balanced focus on exposure and downregulation of emotion is important. So while it is vital to begin to assess the core fears and cognitions, the pace of the sessions must take into account the moment-by-moment emotion regulation of the patient. An additional ally in this process is the recognition that validation by the therapist as well as the chance to express emotions and make sense of experience in a safe interpersonal environment can, in and of themselves, promote emotion regulation and a sense of safety in many patients.

The following case highlights key processes hampering a patient's engagement with the medical team. In addition, challenges to therapeutic engagement are highlighted:

Case Example

Adriana is a 45-year old woman, newly diagnosed with a Stage III ovarian cancer. She had avoided any and all non-emergency medical contact for many years, following what she described as an adverse outcome from a surgical procedure when she was 22. As a young woman, she had needed an emergency appendectomy, which she remembered as painful and frightening, all the more so because she recalled the medical team as having been insensitive, and as having lied to her about the pain she would experience. When she attempted to explain her pain and sought medication, she believed that the doctor scoffed and regarded her as seeking drugs. Adriana was so affected by this experience that she did not obtain a physical for more than 20 years, until the symptoms of what was subsequently revealed to be ovarian cancer could no longer be ignored.

Now, facing a serious medical crisis, Adriana is berating herself for having failed to get help when her cancer might have been detected at an earlier, and potentially more treatable, stage of the illness. She is now facing surgery, possibly followed by radiation therapy and chemotherapy. She becomes increasingly filled with dread as she talks about this in the first session. Her thoughts include "I can't handle this," "I'll go crazy in the hospital," "The doctors don't understand how I can't handle pain." The therapist was aware that missteps in intervening might spark humiliation and rupture the treatment alliance, especially since Adriana was already quite sensitive to being invalidated and misunderstood by caregivers. So the therapist validated her concerns, even her avoidance of routine medical help, in light of her memories of her earlier appendectomy. The therapist was able to communicate an understanding of the logic of Adriana's avoidance, in terms of her history and the current situation, while also helping Adriana begin to address the current need to remain actively engaged with her medical team, and to be committed to dealing with cancer treatment, in the face of her dread.

The processes maintaining Adriana's anxiety vicious cycle include:

1. Experiential avoidance and limited distress tolerance;
2. Underestimation of her ability to manage threat;
3. Self as "weak and helpless";
4. Cognitive biases, including catastrophizing, even though this is clearly a challenging situation for anyone;
5. A limited ability to draw on the medical team as a resource for safety and protection during this ordeal.

Incorporating Psychoeducation into the Treatment Process

In the last chapter, we focused on how to help patients understand how minds work in treating depression and how to normalize their distress. The same strategies apply for anxiety, and for the same reason: many of the patients we see have no prior history with behavioral health professionals, no clear sense of what is going awry, and may be very sensitive to stigmatization. Two key strategies are useful here. First, normalizing fear states, including states of anxious arousal, can help the patient change his or her relationship to fear in ways that foster acceptance and emotion regulation. Second, and in line with teaching people how minds work, the use of direct psychoeducation about anxiety can be supplemented by metaphors and experiential exercises. As was described in Chapter 4 on case formulations, we share the case formulation of the patient's anxiety problems with the patient after we have done sufficient GD/SQ to generate a formulation based on the patient's own experience. If we can map out a vicious cycle of anxiety, including helping the patient see how his or her own efforts to escape are perpetuating the difficulties faced, we can set the stage for interventions to change the pattern. We will address this in case examples later in this chapter.

Metaphors and experiential exercises seem to speak to multiple human information processing systems simultaneously. Since cognition writ large is encoded in verbal, rational modes as well as through imagery, metaphors and exercises are capable of speaking to the head and the gut at the same time. Such interventions can help normalize fear and can ease the way for patients to "befriend" their biologically adaptive threat detection systems, rather than struggle against it. We also want to help ease the possible humiliation inherent in the patient learning that he or she may be employing psychological strategies that are inadvertently maintaining suffering. We used *The Juggler Metaphor* earlier, which is especially apt for anxiety in cancer patients. This metaphor normalizes anxiety in the face of juggling the many challenges that cancer adds to an already full and busy life. Given multiple, and increasing, numbers of items to be juggled in a busy life, added to by the demands of cancer and cancer treatment, it is understandable that worry and anxious arousal increase. The metaphor also highlights the fact that as the number of items to juggle increase, the juggler may be taxed beyond his or her capacity. And as we have described, increasing the capacity of the juggler, the self, is one target of our efforts in treating cancer-related anxiety problems.

Two other metaphors serve as examples of how to help patients begin to normalize the presence of fear, while beginning to address the anxiety equation. This may involve helping the patient achieve clarity about his or her threat estimations, paired with increasing the patient's ability to manage threat. *The Radar Screen Metaphor* can help with the sense of looming vulnerability (Riskind et al., 2012) that can occur in anxiety:

THERAPIST: Imagine that our nervous system is built to include something like a radar screen. We all have one. It's our natural system for detecting dangers in the world and for responding to them. Let's imagine an airman, sitting at an air base, watching a radar screen that is protecting the country, let's say at an Air Force base in Alaska. His job is to watch the screen for incoming missiles and bombers. The radar screen needs to be sensitive, but not too sensitive. The screen and the airman need to be able to pick up on bombers and missiles, but not on sparrows. Imagine that the soldier starts reacting to sparrows on that screen. After a while, the whole Air Force would just be exhausted. What might we say to that airman?

PATIENT: Not everything is dangerous. You've got to figure out which blips to respond to and which ones to let go.

THERAPIST: What if we could figure out some new ways to respond to those blips on your own fear radar screen?

Another metaphor, *The Sentry on the Castle Wall,* can be useful for helping patients befriend their threat detection system, especially if they have been struggling against their fear arousal, including their thoughts, images, and body sensations. This metaphor also can set the stage for experiential interventions to foster self-processes related to managing both threat and anxious arousal:

THERAPIST: Adriana, you've said that you hate these feelings of fear, and the thoughts and images that keep coming up. What if your fear isn't an enemy here, to run from, or fight with? Let's imagine a castle together. It has big walls all around it, and parapets on each corner, with a walkway going all the way around the top of the castle. Imagine for a minute that there's a sentry on the castle wall, patrolling that wall, walking along the walkway at the top of the castle, all the way around the castle, peering out at the forest for any sign of danger out there. Her job is to protect the people inside the castle. So if she does her job, she's going to be exquisitely sensitive to anything that doesn't look right out there. But let's say that she starts to call out "Danger, Danger" every time a leaf blows, or any time the wind parts the brush. On the one hand, she's just doing her job. And on the other, let's imagine that she decides to consult the general inside, before yelling "Danger, Danger" each time she sees something that looks odd. So she quickly climbs down the ladder, goes to the general's chamber, and gets consultation about what she's seen. What if there's a sentry in you, and a general, and we want to help that sentry know when and how to respond to danger, and when and how to take it easy? What if she learned to check with the general in the castle, any time she wasn't sure what to do about what she saw? They're on the same side, and the sentry is just doing her job. She'd just need some help, some training, and the general, like any good general, would want to help. At least that's how it would work in *this* castle.

Dealing with Anxious Cognitive Content

Clinical interventions for anxiety-related cognitions involve targeting both cognitive content and cognitive processes, depending upon which type of cognition is most implicated in anxiety maintenance. Anxiety-related cognitive content can include the same cognitive biases we reviewed in depression and that form the core of Beckian approaches to treatment generally, and to cancer specifically (Moorey & Greer, 2012). It can be a complex and challenging task for the clinician to help patients generate realistic threat estimates of their cancer status. Survival curves speak to averages, not to the individual. Some patients do not want to know about survival prospects. And some physicians do not want to talk about this. Similarly, patients may either harbor overly catastrophic beliefs about treatment or may enter treatment ill prepared for the effects that they will actually experience.

The behavioral health consultant is thus in the position of having to navigate the patient's beliefs, the oncology team's communication styles, and the therapist's own willingness and ability to deal with potentially painful news. As a general rule, I would agree with Levin and Applebaum (2012) that a willingness to engage in best case, median case, and worst case scenarios for prognosis is advisable. In this context, cognitive biases and distortions are more readily apparent and can be addressed.

In the process of exploring anxious cognition, it is especially important to include an assessment of imagery (Hackmann et al., 2011). For example, Caitlin Handley, a 40-year old married mother of two children, in long-term recovery from breast cancer, was being monitored every 6 months. She reported that roughly the week before each visit, her anxiety spiked and she was dogged by a recurrent visual image: she was lying in bed dying, and she peered into the horrified, overwhelmingly sad faces of her children, as they watched her die. In exploring this fear with her, the patient remembered seeing her own father die of cancer when she was 11 years old. Fearing that she, too, would die in the kind of agony she saw her father experience, she was desperately afraid before each monitoring visit that she would learn that she was dying and that her children would suffer as she had when she was 11. This, even more than the sadness of losing them and her husband, and of their losing her, continued to plague her prior to each visit to the oncologist. She noted that it was customary for all her fears to recede immediately after her 6-month monitoring visit with the oncologist, only to recur a week prior to the next visit.

If, using the earlier process, patients maintain realistic estimates of the health threat they face, yet are highly anxious, the therapist can focus on the meaning of the situation to the patient and/or shoring up the patient's coping resources, to manage the threat as effectively as possible. In effect, this targets the numerator and the denominator of the anxiety equation.

Developing a more accurate interpretation of one's circumstances does not necessarily diminish the emotional or behavioral impact of the situation the patient faces. We also need to explore the meaning of those circumstances.

Case Example

Wanda Dooley is 45 and a married mother of two children. She was diagnosed with colon cancer 2 years ago, had surgery and chemotherapy, and was expected to maintain a monitoring schedule consisting of visits to the cancer center every 3 months. She failed to appear for any of the scheduled visits. Now, she returns to the cancer center symptomatic, in pain, and just diagnosed with a recurrence. She faces surgery in 1 week. She is terrified of the recurrence and of the upcoming surgery. In addition, she is blaming herself for the recurrence, because she failed to follow up once in the intervening 2 years. She is convinced that her surgical oncologist is angry with her, and she is equally convinced that she will go crazy from fear and pain after the next surgery, saying, "I won't be able to handle this." If we consider the potential for cognitive biases, we might note that she is jumping to conclusions about both her surgeon and her surgery itself: mind reading involves imagining what others are thinking or feeling, while fortune-telling involves a prediction about the future. It would be heartless to not acknowledge the awfulness of her circumstances; yet there nonetheless remains the likelihood that she is catastrophizing about the surgery. Let's consider each: certainly, in Wanda's case, it is possible that the surgeon is making judgments and is possibly irritated by her failure to adhere to her monitoring following the last surgery he performed on her. She may be right. Yet she may also be exaggerating the extent or reasons for any irritation he might be experiencing and may even be wholly inaccurate about this in the first place. Helping her do some perspective taking about what the physician may or may not be thinking might be useful as an intervention. Helping her find the courage to do the equivalent of a survey technique, by asking the surgeon if he is angry, might also be a useful and important strategy, though perhaps not without risk. At the same time, facing another surgery for her colon cancer is rightfully deeply frightening, and having gone through this before, she is not naïve to the pain and the fear involved for her in enduring this. However, despite the potential grain of truth in each of her automatic thoughts, there is still the prospect of exaggeration and of minimizing her own capacity to tolerate and manage medically necessary interventions. As we can see, both parts of the anxiety equation are worthy of exploration, since our task will be to help her both deal with the surgeon and the surgery.

Clinical strategies for Wanda Dooley might include helping her recognize that she is both assuming the worst of the surgery and of her coping abilities. The automatic thought "I'll go crazy" was explored in some detail. Underneath "I'll go crazy" was the concern "I'll alienate the staff," and this, in turn, seemed to rest on her fear of being alone, misunderstood, and in pain while recovering from the surgery. She was afraid that she would simply not be able to deal with the pain, and this, in turn, connected with her sense that she had not had adequate pain management following the last surgery:

THERAPIST: Could you tell me a little more about going crazy.

WANDA: Oh, I'd just go completely crazy, and they wouldn't want to see that on the inpatient unit.

THERAPIST: What would going crazy actually look like? I mean, if I could see you going absolutely at your imagined worst, what would it look like?

WANDA: Well, you'd see and hear me yelling. I'd be yelling and cursing because I'd be in pain, and nobody would be coming to help me. Or the nurse would show up, like last time, and would say "The doctor didn't authorize any additional medication for your pain."

THERAPIST: OK. So it sounds like you'd be really angry, right? I mean, the picture I'm getting is that you'd be angry.

WANDA: Way over the top angry!

THERAPIST: Well, that's certainly possible. But I'm also imagining you in that hospital bed after surgery. And it sounds like you're also scared. Scared about being in pain and not having anyone on the team willing or able to understand and help you? (This would be a Level 3 Validation strategy in DBT.)

WANDA: Yes. That's exactly what happened last time. And if I get mad at them this time, it'll push them even farther away. And I'll get *no* help whatsoever.

THERAPIST: OK. I can see why you're concerned about getting angry at them. So you're scared. And you're afraid you'll get mad and yell.

WANDA: And they'll just think I'm this drug-seeking crazy woman. I can't handle that!

THERAPIST: Well, suppose we could figure out some ways to do some advance planning with the staff and the docs about this, so they understand and we all help you manage your pain after surgery?

The grain of truth in her concerns was managed via problem solving with her surgeon and the team, in advance of her surgery. Her own distress tolerance and pain tolerance abilities were targeted as well. This included helping her connect to what purposes and values were served by going through the surgery and what potential benefits awaited her and her family once she recovered. Both Beckian CBT and ACT recognize that fear is at times an inherent part of the human condition. We can't think it away, and this is especially true in situations such as Wanda's. Even with accurate threat estimates, one still may require great courage to face the threat. The ACT model can inform our efforts in this regard, by helping us target the patient's ability and willingness to experience fear, while encouraging the patient to engage in purposeful behavior. We will return to Wanda's case later in this chapter, to address her avoidance of follow-up.

Wells identified two forms of worry (Wells, 2009). One, called Type I worry, is essentially the worry that humans are heir to. With cancer patients, Type I worry can take a huge array of forms: worry about the prospects of dying, about disfigurement, sexual diminishment, loss of important roles, pain management, fatigue, and so forth. Cognitive interventions for worry may focus on the accuracy or inaccuracy of the patient's appraisals as well as the hidden meanings that sometimes lie behind even the fear of death. For example, for some, the stated fear of death is really about a fear of dying in pain. Working with patients and their medical teams to manage pain can thus diminish the actual threat that is greatest to the patient. Thus, our efforts with the cognitive content of worry involve two things: helping with threat assessments and helping to problem solve and cope, once we have an understanding of patient appraisals.

Addressing the Process of Worry

In dealing with worry in cancer patients, the clinician needs to be vigilant for when to address the content of worry versus dealing with worry as a process. Recursive, endless worry, amplified by metacognitive beliefs about worry's danger or efficacy, suggests the need to target worry as a process. Wells identified what he referred to as Type II worry (Wells, 2009), which involves beliefs in either the efficacy of worry ("Worry is useful to me. If I stop worrying, bad things will happen.") or beliefs that worry is dangerous and out of control ("If I keep worrying like this, I will go crazy" or "Worry will cause my cancer to spread like wildfire."). The latter, which includes metacognitive beliefs that worry is dangerous, seem especially implicated in cancer-related distress (Cook et al., 2015). Borkovec (2006) postulated that worry, chiefly verbally mediated worry, serves an avoidant function, by reducing one's exposure to painful emotions. The more the person worries, the lower the anxious arousal can become, but at the price of maintaining a chronic level of anxiety. Hayes, Villatte et al. (2011) described efforts to control and eliminate painful internal experience as a maintaining factor in anxiety disorders, suggesting that efforts to control thoughts is not a solution; it is among the problems. In contrast, Wells said that control is the solution, not the problem, as long as the right kind of control is exerted over the process of problematic worry (Wells, 2009).

Although the theories and philosophies of science differ in these models, there is a convergence with regards to what to do with problematic worry. The first step out of entrapment in worry is deceptively simple: enter the present moment. Thomas Borkovec, a leading GAD researcher, stated, "There can be no anxiety or depression in the present moment" (State of Mind, 2012). This dovetails with the focus of other mindfulness and acceptance-based CBT models, all of which emphasize that worry and rumination occur when the mind is focused on either the past or the future. Strategies that gently help the patient direct attention and awareness to the present can free the patient of intense levels of worry and rumination and open the moment for engagement in areas of other areas life.

Opening up to the present moment by no means necessarily reduces fear, and in cancer care we don't rid people of fear. We foster present moment, mindful awareness, in a way that allows fear to be present, while also fostering resilient self-processes, bolstering the anxiety equation denominator. Cancer sparks fear. Cancer therapies spark fear. So do the uncertainties about the future that cancer incites. It is the inability to shift modes, or self-states, that is problematic. It is the incessant stoking of the threat system, via the transdiagnostic maintaining processes in this book, which is the problem we target. Our therapeutic aim is the reduction of suffering and increased cognitive and behavioral flexibility in the face of cancer's threats, not the eradication of fear itself. If our inner radar screen identifies bombers and incoming rockets, we mobilize resources to deal with them. When sparrows spark fear, we can pause mindfully in the present, to take stock and choose accordingly.

Clinical Strategies for Worry

Interventions for Type II worry involve altering attentional processes, fostering an observer stance toward one's internal processes, and fostering flexible engagement in the opportunities and demands of the moment. The ability to be flexible in one's attention deployment, while remaining mindfully in the present moment, is a skill to cultivate in addressing chronic worry. Given the brevity of many of our therapy encounters, we need to focus on selectively and prescriptively targeting relevant processes and creating moments in session that are experientially compelling and relevant.

Metacognitive Interventions

Patients with an overblown sense of the importance of worry can be asked to walk through the pros and cons of engaging in worry. It is quite possible that the patient has not considered the cons of worry. Using a sheet of paper to encourage the patient to list pros and cons and to provide a rating at the end can help reduce the sense that worry is important. For example, it may be possible for a patient who begins with a strong conviction that worry is necessary, to conclude, after reviewing in detail the pros and cons, that the balance has shifted from 100% pro, to something like 30% to 70% con. Yet even when patients come to see that chronic worry is a relatively useless activity, they may still be hard pressed to alter their engagement in worry. This can link with another form of Type II worry, the belief that one's mind is spinning dangerously out of control. And this, too, links with the previous discussion about when control is the problem and which type of control is indicated when. ACT defusion exercises, of the sort we reviewed in treating depression, can be utilized to help people change their stance toward worry, and to alter its function. Ironically, by giving up the effort to control the mind, a more benign and functional control can emerge. The patient can be invited to consider whether, in fact, their mind is engaged in worry constantly, and under what conditions worry processes are not present. This, in turn, can spark the awareness that worry is neither completely uncontrollable nor particularly dangerous. Wells's MCT model uses a modified form of Socratic Questioning to address both positive and negative metacognitions (Type II worry). For example, the belief that worry is important or useful can be addressed via reattribution interventions, such as analyzing the pros and cons, earlier, or by reducing the patient's conviction that prolonged engagement in worry is important or useful (Wells, 2009). Here is an example:

THERAPIST: Do you believe that you must spend hours a day focusing on your body, to make sure that your cancer isn't back?

PATIENT: I didn't pay attention last time when I had a small lump. I waited too long, and when I went in, I was already Stage II. I can't afford that again. So, yes, I suppose I do think that I need to be very tuned in.

THERAPIST: How many hours a day do you spend now, worrying and scanning your body for signs that something is wrong?

PATIENT: Depends. For sure, when I get closer to coming in for a scan, and follow-up, I probably start worrying a lot, and yes, I spend maybe 2 to 4 hours a day like this?

THERAPIST: And what happens while this is going on, as far as your body and emotions?

PATIENT: Oh, I am just beside myself with worry. I'm a mess. I'm absolutely miserable.

THERAPIST: But a *necessary* mess, right? In other words, if you didn't spend all this time focusing on your body like this, you'd what?

PATIENT: Miss something, I guess.

THERAPIST: Would it serve your interests to spend less time on this? Even, say, 20 minutes or so? What do you think? Will you actually be safer if you spend hours focusing on your body and becoming miserable?

PATIENT: No. I'll still be scared, though, until my follow-up visit is over, and Dr. Smith tells me I'm OK.

THERAPIST: So you'll have some fear no matter what, right? How about some fear, minus some misery?

PATIENT: That would be a tradeoff I can learn to live with.

Reattribution techniques for the other form of Type II worry, the belief that worry is uncontrollable or dangerous, are also warranted (Wells, 2009). The aim is to help people recognize that their beliefs about worry as dangerous and uncontrollable are not literally accurate. For example, one technique that can be employed is that of *scheduling worry time*. By acknowledging that worry has its place, the patient is encouraged to designate specific times and places for full and complete engagement in worry. Using an activity schedule sheet, this can be done to help highlight the possibility that even marginal control is possible, which, too, violates the rule that worry is uncontrollable. In addition, finding other times in the patient's day when worry is not present can help reduce the impact of metacognitive beliefs:

THERAPIST: So you're scared that your mind is spinning out of control? That you can't stop worrying? Ever?

PATIENT: Yes. Cancer is always on my mind. I am always imagining it's back, even after the doctor says I'm clear. I know I am clear; but it's my mind that's driving me mad now.

THERAPIST: Are there exceptions, any times when you don't think your mind is driving you mad?

PATIENT: What do you mean?

THERAPIST: Let's go back over the week for a moment. Was there a time, any time, when you weren't worrying?

PATIENT: (Silently thinking about the past week) Well, when I was with my granddaughter, for a while I was just laughing and having fun with her.

THERAPIST: I see. Great. Where was "I have cancer" then?

PATIENT: Not in the neighborhood.

These types of exceptions, of which there are likely many that the patient is overlooking, help the patient learn that his or her belief in uncontrollable worry is not literally true. Similarly, beliefs that worry can cause or exacerbate cancer may also need to be addressed in therapy. While it is certainly true that prolonged states of chronic stress arousal can affect immune functioning, and impacts health status in some ways, there is no evidence supporting the notion that stress and/or worry cause or exacerbate cancer. And it is also not literally true that worry is dangerously out of control. The more one struggles against it, the more it's there. Both MCT and ACT recognize the importance of stopping the struggle and focusing on what matters. Each model, though, provides differing accounts and technologies for accomplishing these objectives.

Attention Training

Metacognitive Therapy includes The Attention Training Technique and Detached Mindfulness (Wells, 2009) as techniques for addressing worry and rumination. Flexible control over the deployment of attention is a foundational human skill. It is an initial intervention target in virtually all mindfulness programs (Kabat-Zinn, 2013; Segal et al., 2013). Sonja Lyubomirsky, a leading scientist in the Positive Psychology movement, quoted William James, who wrote, "My experience is what I agree to attend to. Only those items which I notice shape my mind." Lyubomirsky added that "this idea—which is really mind-boggling when we think about it—suggests that *our life experience is that on which we choose to focus* [emphasis added]" (Lyubomirsky, 2013). The Attention Training Technique (ATT) in Metacognitive Therapy is intended to rather quickly and simply help the patient direct his or her awareness from internal processes to external stimuli. Sound, in particular, has been found to be a powerful stimulus for directing attention (Wells, 2009). Training can be done in short increments of time, and practice sessions can be done through the use of recordings made in the office that the patient takes home. Ten minutes of ATT in session may be sufficient to help produce a heightened sense of attentional control; Wells was careful to note, in line with ACT, that this must be done in a way that does not shore up experiential avoidance. In other words, attention training is about flexible attention, directed toward "that on which we choose to focus," not on running in fear from uncontrollable or dangerous thoughts, or on preoccupation with remote and potentially implausible dangers (Wells, 2009).

Tolerating Uncertainty

Intolerance of uncertainty is common in chronic worry. And uncertainty is a constant companion on the cancer journey: uncertainty about outcome, about recurrence prospects, about treatment side effects, about how others will view one, about the impact of cancer on one's work life, one's social network, one's energy and stamina, one's sexual functioning. And ultimately, uncertainty about survival always looms on the journey. In terms of the anxiety equation, our treatment efforts involve helping patients live with the uncertainty of the outcome, in all areas affected by cancer. Leahy (2006) provided strategies for helping people practice uncertainty tolerance. These include acceptance of reality as well as allowing oneself to feel the emotions that are present in the situation. As we have reviewed earlier, bringing in imagery and emotion allows the patient to process core fears in a way that promotes problem solving where that is possible and acceptance where problem solving is a limited tool. Conducting a cost-benefit analysis of tolerating uncertainty can also be helpful. Linehan's (1993a; 2015) ideas about Radical Acceptance are powerful and useful here as well. DBT teaches that reality acceptance and uncertainty tolerance do not necessarily occur by an act of will, in one sudden and permanent epiphany. Both can involve "Turning the Mind" over and over, as a commitment that must be lived and practiced, possibly over the course of a lifetime. The alternative to Radical Acceptance can be a life of misery.

Intolerance of uncertainty represents a form of non-acceptance. In turn, it can involve a lack of conviction in one's ability to manage difficulties when they arise.

Case Example

Lynn McMahon is a 34-year-old violinist, who is experiencing mild neuropathy following multiple courses of chemotherapy for breast cancer. She is noticing that her violin playing speed and accuracy is affected. Because of the level of her performance standards, and the complexity of her repertoire, she is deeply worried that "I will never be able to play in concert again." "I have to know whether my hands will come back," she adds.

THERAPIST: Is that knowable now?

PATIENT: No. My doctor said it might be months before I will know. But I can't stand that. I can't stand having to wait like this!

THERAPIST: Is there another option here?

PATIENT: (Smiles) No. But I don't like that.

THERAPIST: OK, well, let's say the options are: one, you get your hands back; two, you don't. I'm with you in hoping for you to get your full hand use back. Suppose not, though. What would that mean to you?

PATIENT: It would mean a big part of my life is over. Having an audience who appreciates my playing means so much to me. (Eyes well with tears)

THERAPIST: What are your tears saying?

PATIENT: Just sadness, just a terrible sadness.

THERAPIST: Lynn, I'm really hoping you can get back up on that stage with a symphony or a chamber group again. If you can't, can you trust yourself to find a way through? To still have a life that matters to you?

PATIENT: (Silence). I'd rather not have to face that.

THERAPIST: I hope you don't face it. And, if that's what's in the cards, could you do it?

PATIENT: You know, I could, I suppose. I just don't want to.

THERAPIST: And in the meantime, you're playing these days, right?

PATIENT: Yes. I practice. I play lullabies for my little girl. She falls asleep sometimes to my playing.

THERAPIST: So you have an appreciative audience, even now!

PATIENT: Yeah. I guess I do. I don't want grownups to fall asleep when I play.
(Laughs)

THERAPIST: So we can't know for a good long while what life will give you, in
terms of the neuropathy in your hands. Time will tell. In the meantime, you can play, and it sure sounds to me that there's something
lovely that happens for your little girl when you play for her at night.
Will she and your husband love and appreciate you, even if your playing is always the way it is right now?

PATIENT: Yes. And for now, at least, maybe that's all I need.

Present Moment Mindfulness Practices

A creative and exciting area for individual CBT with cancer patients is the inclusion of mindfulness practices. These can help promote experiential entry into
the present moment. Ideally, cancer patients would be involved in an MBSR or
MBCT program while undergoing cancer therapy. As we have discussed, that
is often not feasible, due to time and energy demands as well as the effects of
the illness. In addition, many patients referred to a behavioral health clinician
are in a state of acute distress (Levin & Applebaum, 2012), which necessitates
a brief and highly focused therapy encounter. Nonetheless, the therapist who
is skilled in incorporating ACT, DBT, and/or MBCT practices into therapy can
provide moments to pause from suffering. These moments provide experiential evidence to patients that their lives needn't be dominated by cancer at all
times and that it is possible in the midst of pain and suffering to notice the
moment, with its richness. In addition, exercises such as MBCT's 3-minute
breathing space can be employed to help patients achieve grounding in the
midst of intense distress as well as for more traditional exposure work, as indicated by the patient's needs. I customarily employ multi-sensory experiential
processes during relatively brief exercises, lasting no more than 10–12 minutes,
as the patient and his or her companions may tolerate. A sample script was
presented in Chapter 6 on treating depression in cancer patients, and includes
the following:

1.   Entering a posture conducive to abdominal breathing and a sense of
dignity;
2.   Tuning in to sounds in the room, and other sensory experiences;
3.   Noticing the flight of thoughts that emerge inevitably, non-judgmentally,
and with curiosity and compassion;
4.   Allowing awareness to return to sensory experience;

5. Bringing awareness to the breath, with guided instructions in regards to abdominal breathing and pace;
6. Returning to the room to discuss any reactions or experiences of the exercise.

Fostering Distress Tolerance

Many of the patients with whom we work, especially those in acute distress, require strategies for rapid regulation of intense emotions. There are discussions in the treatment literature regarding the use of safety, or avoidance behaviors, in conducting exposures (Deacon et al., 2010; Levy & Radomsky, 2014). The debate centers on when safety behaviors may serve to bolster experiential avoidance and when they may promote engagement in exposures. For many of our cancer patients, there is no luxury to titrate exposure to fear-evoking stimuli. Cancer, alas, can create one long dive into a pool of fear-evoking stimuli. In such cases, DBT distress tolerance and self-soothing skills can be incorporated with good effect into individual, couple, or even family sessions. Although DBT was developed for patients with severe emotion and behavior dysregulation problems, chiefly those with borderline personality disorder, these skills are potentially highly useful for managing distress overload in cancer patients. Using our anxiety equation, one can see that strengthening the capacity to tolerate and manage distress is one way to shift the equation. Distress tolerance skills may be delivered using a mindfulness practice of noticing the moment, though without necessarily a focus on the breath or on any internal processes. Highly distressed patients may have a limited capacity for these more internal foci of attention and thus may be more responsive to sensory processes. DBT's mindfulness skills involve being able to observe, to describe, and to notice when judgments versus facts come into the mind. The patient is given a mini training in these skills, and it is applied in simple, accessible ways, through multiple sensory modalities.

Visual

Find a spot in the consulting room to bring your eyes to and to notice. Bring full awareness to the area in the room, and see if you can pay attention with some gentle curiosity, as though you have never seen this before. Describe, in your mind, the shapes and colors, as though this is the first time you have noticed this, and do not have a word for it, a name. Just noticing.

The patient(s) can then talk after the exercise about what was noticed, from a place of describing, not judging.

The therapist can lead exercises involving other visual stimuli: the back of the hand in the light through a window; the texture, shape, colors of a ball; a vase or art object in the consulting room; a lava lamp.

Auditory

Attention can be brought to sounds, including soothing or pleasant music; the sound of a stream or a waterfall accessed through the Internet. The patient can be encouraged to help generate a list of potentially engaging, pleasant sounds to access in session and to practice at home.

Tactile

Self-administered hand massages can be practiced in session. Lotion can be applied. Patients and therapist can both practice the skill in session, with the therapist providing a verbal guide to the practice. I tend to include a wide net of experiences in the hand massage: finding the hand that needs attention the most; finding the finger(s) that can deliver the attention; finding spots that are sweet spots; experimenting with massage over the entire hand, including all fingers, the palm, the base of the palm, the back of the hand; varying pressure and noticing differences.

Smell and Taste

Because smell and taste are linked and can both be affected by cancer treatment, I encourage proceeding with mild caution with these, especially if the therapist knows that the patient has had a loss or unpleasant alteration of taste, due to cancer and/or cancer therapies. Nonetheless, if this area of sensory experience is relatively unimpaired, it, too, can provide a good entry point into the present moment and into distress tolerance. Finally, along these lines, it can be useful for the patient to make sensory contact with the sensory object as it is experienced, with altered smell and taste, or absent taste, if the patient is willing to do so. This may not only help with distress tolerance, it can help foster reality acceptance and can de-catastrophize the changes in sensory experience. Clinical sensitivity and tact must guide the decision about this. Aromatherapy can be helpful. One patient remembered a rose-scented perfume that her grandmother wore when the patient was a child. She bought a rose-scented perfume that evoked pleasant memories of her beloved late grandmother and kept it with her for use during the day, and while in clinic. Not only did the scent promote self-soothing and enhance distress tolerance, it also evoked the memory presence of her grandmother, a source of strength in the patient's early life.

The Raisin Exercise is borrowed from Kabat-Zinn (2013) and Segal et al. (2013). It involves placing a raisin into the patient's hand while the patient's eyes are initially closed. The patient is encouraged to bring full awareness to the raisin, visually, tactilely, through smell, and finally through a long, lingering experience of taste. Bringing the mind of a curious child to the experience can evoke a sense of "first time ever" to the raisin, which most patients have eaten rapidly, by the handful, and without awareness for much of their lives. Younger patients may enjoy intensely sweet and sour candies, though, again, the therapist must assess first whether taste and smell are impaired, and what impact might occur if the exercise is pursued.

Linking Mindfulness and Distress Tolerance Skills to Exposure Work

We can incorporate DBT mindfulness and distress tolerance skills into imaginal exposure by encouraging patients to notice judgments versus descriptions of experiences involving cancer and cancer therapy. In addition, we can create imaginal exposures to upcoming, fear-evoking procedures, or other stimuli, such as waiting for the results of a test. By doing this, we can help patients access judgments that predispose them toward catastrophizing ("I'll go crazy from fear while I'm waiting to get the CT scan results"), versus something like "I'll be scared as hell, but I've done this before, and I'll handle it no matter what I hear." In addition, cognitive, distress tolerance, and problem-solving skills can be utilized to help bridge imaginal exposure and the target situations that evoke fear for the patient.

Self-Processes

Perspective-taking skills can be employed using guided imagery and experiential exercises for anxiety, as in the treatment of depression. These exercises address the anxiety equation by helping the patient access the strengths and resources that have fueled their life journey during other challenging times. Perspective-taking exercises can also be one way of helping patients contact wise and compassionate self-states. There is evidence demonstrating that states of lovingkindness and compassion impact overall well-being (Gilbert & Choden, 2014; Tirch et al., 2014). There is also emerging evidence suggesting that CBT can be enhanced by fostering states of lovingkindness and compassion, rather than focusing primarily on removing depressive and anxious cognition (Hofmann, 2011; Hofmann et al., 2015). Some patients may be tragically blocked, by virtue of their developmental histories, from experiencing self-compassion. Incorporation of techniques from Compassion Focused Therapy (Gilbert, 2009a; Tirch et al., 2014) can strengthen the clinician's ability to deliver effective experiential exercises. MBCT's focus on being mode and doing mode dovetails, in the sense that modes of being involve accessing and practicing self-states. Brief, focused experiential exercises can help tilt the anxiety equation toward a greater sense of strength in the face of adversity. It is quite possible that the primary vehicle for fostering self-compassion in cancer patients is via the therapist. MBCT appears to increase self-compassion, with the model provided by the therapist as perhaps the key vehicle (Segal et al., 2013).

A more traditional CBT focus can also be employed to help people access and build resilient self-processes (Kuyken et al., 2009; Padesky & Mooney, 2012; Bennett-Levy et al., 2015). These methods employ a more rationalist style of intervention than a guided imagery focus, yet they also are experiential. And they, like the ACT and CFT interventions, lead to action, by helping the patient engage in meaningful activities, and with people, rather than remaining embroiled in states of distress.

There are not treatment outcome studies comparing these approaches with one another, to provide clear guidelines for clinicians working with cancer patients. I would offer some thoughts and would encourage clinicians to adopt an experimental approach: see what works. When the number of sessions is limited, as it often is in cancer centers, it may well be worth using guided experiential exercises in an effort to rapidly access healing self-states; this could involve helping people access their repertoire of resilient coping behaviors and bring them to bear on managing the challenges posed by cancer. Kuyken et al. (2009) suggested strategies for assessing patient strengths by using Guided Discovery and Socratic Questioning to find areas of strength in the patient's life. When working with cancer patients for whom cancer has taken over their life, it is possible to use these strategies to help patients recall and connect with times in their lives when strengths were readily apparent. The perspective-taking exercises we employed in Chapter 6, with depression, target similar processes. Helping cancer patients connect, or re-connect, with these strengths and values can help tilt the anxiety equation in favor of moving forward with fear as a passenger, rather than as the driver (Hayes, Strosahl, & Wilson, 2012).

Case Example

Let's return to the case of Wanda Dooley, who refused cancer monitoring for 2 years, prior to her recurrence, and who again faces the recommendation of every 3-month monitoring. Wanda's vicious cycle of avoidance is shown in Figure 7.1.

Wanda was able to recognize that the payoff of avoidance was a rapid drop in anxiety. If she simply didn't show up for follow-up visits, she didn't have to face her fear of recurrence. Short term, her avoidance worked effectively to blockade anxiety. But Wanda also realized that the longer term consequences of avoidance were potentially devastating: untreated recurrence and an increased likelihood of death. Using Bennett-Levy et al.'s (2015) model, we were able to help identify values and strengths, including Wanda's love of her family, and her wish to be present at future life cycle events for her children. This, in turn, helped reframe follow-up visits in terms of a different purpose. In Wanda's case, the purpose of going through the pain, fear, and uncertainty of follow-up visits was to protect not only her life but also her future chances to be there for her children and husband. Humans can endure enormous pain, if it is purposeful (Yalom, 1980; Frankl, 1986; 1992; Hayes, Strosahl, & Wilson, 2012). Helping Wanda connect to those purposes and values will potentially help her follow through on the decision to monitor her cancer status every 3 months, for the rest of her life, if need be. Wanda and the therapist addressed each cognitive, emotional, and behavioral barrier to change, which appears in the avoidance cycle in Figure 7.1. By focusing on "new ways of being"

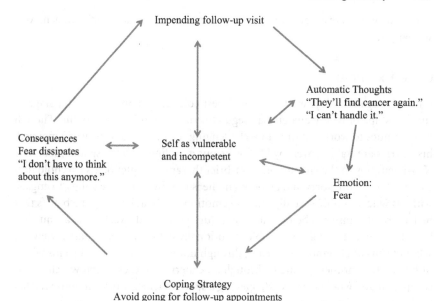

FIGURE 7.1 Vicious Cycle: Wanda Dooley

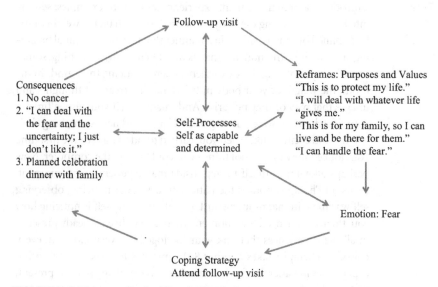

FIGURE 7.2 Virtuous Cycle: Wanda Dooley

(Bennett-Levy et al., 2015), a fresh pattern was constructed, to support medical adherence, not out of a perceived need to comply with doctor's orders, but from a place of personal meaning and purpose. This new way of being, or virtuous cycle, is shown in Figure 7.2.

Following is an example of how to employ an experiential exercise to achieve a similar purpose.

Case Example

Carlos Ortega is a 35-year-old man with testicular cancer, in the re-entry stage of survivorship, for whom anxiety has begun to crowd out other areas of life. Though he continues to work full time in a challenging tech career and is newly married, his worries are "taking over my life," as he put it. In line with the spatial metaphor we will employ in the chapter on ultra-brief therapy, Chapter 8, his psychological room is filled with worry and anxiety, and he is rapidly losing the ability to engage with his wife, not only sexually but also emotionally. In addressing the beliefs that he has about himself as being "damaged," "unmanly," and "weak," one avenue has been through searching for credible, emotionally compelling alternative views of self, in terms of generating evidence, through not only his eyes, but also his wife's, of his worth. Another avenue is through an experiential exercise, in which self as competent and whole is accessed, opening a space in which work can more readily be done to identify strengths, and to set a course for re-engagement in life.

THERAPIST: (Introduces a present moment experience, as in prior examples: settling into the chair, noticing the body contoured to the chair, the weight of the body pulled by gravity, sitting in a manner that fosters abdominal breathing and dignity) And noticing that as we sit here, now, something, someone within is noticing these experiences here. Noticing the sounds in the room, the weight of your body in the chair, the stream of thoughts and images that may or may not arise. And imagining, if you wish, a time in your life when you were learning something brand new, something challenging and exciting, like when you learned to ride a bike, or the first time you noticed how many cool things you could do on the computer. Now perhaps allowing yourself to step inside that experience for a moment. (Pause) (Therapist notices the patient smiles) That noticing, observing self was there in that moment, just as that observing self is noticing how you, then, experienced that moment, then. You've been a steady presence in all the experiences that link your life together, every moment, every episode (Therapist takes another 8–10 minutes to walk through other experiences in patient's life where an observing, noticing self was present, up to and including the current time, in his dealings with cancer)

When the therapist and patient conclude the exercise, they talk about the experience of viewing life from the place of an observing presence that links episodes of a life together into a consistent, coherent whole. The therapist and patient focused on the experience from his earlier life that had come to mind: a moment when, at about age 10, he became enchanted by computer technology. It was a moment that kindled a sense of curiosity and wonder. Connecting to the zest for life inside that experience helped set the stage for Carlos access those strengths in his current challenge. The therapist focused with Carlos on how, specifically, those strengths and values might show up in the present, and what behaviors might link them to his daily life, with his wife, and with his job.

We will conclude the chapter with two extended case studies.

Extended Case Studies

A Case of Panic

Carl Ferguson is a 47-year-old married father of adult twin daughters. A naso-pharyngeal cancer required surgery, which resulted in his throat being cut open, except for a small area just over the larynx. The incision ran otherwise across the entire width of the throat, nearly from ear to ear. With no prior history of anxiety disorders, and one prior history of a depressive episode, Mr. Ferguson became anxious just after diagnosis, and was prescribed an anxiolytic, Loraze-pam, to help him cope with the demanding and frightening procedures he faced. Just weeks after surgery, Mr. Ferguson began noticing tightening sensations in the throat. The sensation ran the length of the surgical scar and seemed to center on the area that had not been cut, just over the larynx. He interpretation the sen-sation as that of clamping down, and he experienced both thoughts and mental images of choking. He had the automatic thoughts "I can't breathe" and "I am choking," which were accompanied by panic episodes, which he had never expe-rienced before. These sensations, along with panic, meant to him "I am dying," which further exacerbated his panic. He found that he was able to manage these episodes, which were increasing in frequency, by rotating his neck and head to relieve the sensation, and by taking Lorazepam. His case conceptualization appears in Figure 7.3.

Figure 7.3 displays a vicious cycle of anxiety, showing how panic is conceptual-ized in CBT (D.M. Clark, 1986; Butler et al., 2008). Clark's model of panic disorder specifies that panic disorder is driven by a catastrophic interpretation of a benign body sensation. Such thoughts as "I am dying" and "I'm having a stroke" reflect an imminent sense of danger in panic disorder. By contrast, health anxiety, which is conceptually similar to panic disorder, is customarily conceptualized as interpre-tations of bodily sensations in anticipation of a future threat of illness (Salkovskis, 1996a; Butler et al., 2008). Carl Ferguson's throat sensations were experienced in the moment as posing an imminent threat of death. In contrast to the customary presentation of panic, Mr. Ferguson's physical sensations could easily be seen as anything but benign. His throat had been cut nearly ear-to-ear in an effort to save him from the cancer, leaving pain, scarring, and difficulty swallowing. The thera-pist explored Mr. Ferguson's knowledge about the nature of his surgical recovery and whether he had expressed his fears to his oncology or surgical teams. He had not. The therapist encouraged Mr. Ferguson and the team to talk directly about the sensation in Mr. Ferguson's throat and about his fears. He was provided reas-surance by his surgeon that the tightening sensation he felt, and the pressure across

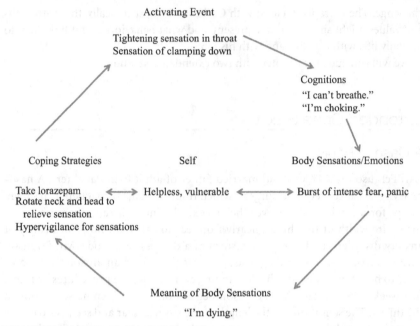

Activating Event

Tightening sensation in throat
Sensation of clamping down

Cognitions
"I can't breathe."
"I'm choking."

Coping Strategies   Self   Body Sensations/Emotions

Take lorazepam ⟷ Helpless, vulnerable ⟷ Burst of intense fear, panic
Rotate neck and head to
  relieve sensation
Hypervigilance for sensations

Meaning of Body Sensations

"I'm dying."

FIGURE 7.3 Vicious Cycle: Carl Ferguson

the larynx area, was simply the healing process, following surgery. Despite these assurances that his airway was not closing, and that he was not choking, Mr. Ferguson continued to struggle with panic episodes. As is often the case in panic disorder, the brain versus gut split occurred: in session, Mr. Ferguson was able to state with 90% certainty that he was not dying in these episodes, yet once the tightening sensation and clamping down sensation started, his insight fled, and he became equally certain that he was dying. He felt trapped and helpless by the seeming irrationality of his fear, yet unable to manage them easily when panic occurred. He was beginning to spend increasing amounts of time each day mentally checking his airway to insure that he was breathing adequately. And he was starting to limit his daily range of activities just in case he had an airway emergency.

The panic vicious cycle, shown in Figure 7.3 was drawn in session and shown to him. He was asked if there were any elements in the cycle that he would amend. There were not. The following vignette demonstrates cognitive interventions, especially targeting the avoidance, or safety behaviors he was employing as a means of creating an alternative explanation.

THERAPIST: I am noticing here (points to vicious cycle sheet) that this cycle comes to an end, at least for a while, when you either rotate your head and neck, or take a Lorazepam. Is that right?

CARL: Yes. That's what happens. When it starts, it's like I've got a clamp down, right over my throat (Shows therapist, by putting thumb over throat)

THERAPIST: This was actually the one area that was *not* cut during the surgery, though, right?

CARL: Yes. The surgeon said the scar tissue is pulling as it heals, and I'm feeling a little tightening over the larynx. If I turn my head like this (demonstrates) and turn my neck, it eases up. If that doesn't work right away, I take a Lorazepam, and it seems that in a few minutes things settle down.

THERAPIST: What do you make of the fact that the Lorazepam helps with this? Does that support the idea that you are dying when this happens?

CARL: Well, no. Lorazepam isn't an effective treatment for an airway that's closing down. Like the surgeon said, the scar tissue is healing, and it's pulling a little. When I rotate my neck, maybe it loosens up the tissue a little bit. But boy, when it happens, I just panic. And it scares the hell out of my wife, too. Then I can't get my mind off this thing, and even when it's not happening, I'm starting to check, like we said, all the time, to see if my throat is OK. It's driving me nuts. And I don't go anywhere without a bottle of Lorazepam.

THERAPIST: OK. So one theory about this is that when you feel this tightening, it means you're choking to death. Another theory here might be the one your surgeon suggested. The tightening sensation means you are actually healing up from the surgical scars.

CARL: Yeah. The second theory is probably correct. But I have to convince myself of that when it's happening.

The therapeutic task was to break up the panic cycle at the earliest point in the cycle at which attention could be brought to bear. Therapy involved activating the sensation, and the core fears, including the most emotionally salient, hot cognitions and images, by stimulating the sensation of his throat clamping down. He was able to do this manually, by gently pulling the skin behind the surgical scars, slightly increasing pressure over the larynx. He was asked to allow the sensations, the thoughts, and the emotions to remain present, without fighting them and without using or having Lorazepam in his pocket. The duration of the exposure did not require a specific reduction in distress. Mr. Ferguson said afterward that during the first exposure he was able to restore normal breathing and to notice the cascade of thoughts and fear sensations while his breathing spontaneously normalized. Controlled breathing is not generally advised as a treatment strategy for dealing with panic, due to the possibility that breath control can become an avoidance, or safety, behavior. In debriefing after the exposure, he had, in fact, not used safety, or avoidance, behaviors he had previously been using, including Lorazepam.

Mr. Ferguson took the written Panic Vicious Cycle (Figure 7.3) with him. He agreed to notice when the tightening sensation occurred in his throat and to allow it to be there, noticing the fear and the thoughts that his breathing was shutting down. The brain versus gut phenomenon, in which multiple modes of information processing can compete with one another, was evident in Mr. Ferguson's panic exposures. He became increasingly able to trust "Theory 2," which said that the sensations signified that his surgical scar was healing, rather than closing down. Once more fully healed, the panic, too, dissipated. The patient went on to a new round of therapy, radiation therapy.

The previous case demonstrates not only how to work with the content of panic beliefs but also how to do so in a way that targets multiple modes of information processing and that occurs in the context of engagement in exposure situations. We used the most salient and parsimonious principles and techniques to target the panic presentation in as rapid a manner as feasible. In addition, the patient was able to benefit rapidly in part because the panic presentation was based on adjustment to a surgical intervention and had not developed into full-blown panic disorder, including with agoraphobia.

A Case of PTSD Following Cancer Treatment

Let's return to the case of Liz Romano, age 26, from the Introduction. Nearly one year out from two brain surgeries, followed by radiation therapy for a rare cancerous tumor of the skull, she was experiencing increased anxiety, accompanied by puzzling and disturbing experiences. Each time she had a headache, she interpreted it to mean that her cancer had returned. Even more disturbing were the intense and vivid re-living experiences that spontaneously began soon after the completion of treatment. She spontaneously and unpredictably experienced the physical sensations that occurred upon awakening from anesthetic and her first brain surgery. She felt and imagined searing pain, radiating from her head, down her spine. She spontaneously re-experienced the feelings and the images of vomiting up blood. This replay was increasing in frequency, and she was at a loss to understand what was happening. She has never told anyone else about this.

The therapist used GD/SQ to elicit in detail the experiences of re-living. Mrs. Romano quickly was able to establish a trusting relationship and had a strong history of adaptive functioning as well as both strong psychological and interpersonal resources. Following is a sample transcript of how the PTSD cycle was elicited.

THERAPIST: Liz, can you walk me through what happens, almost like I'm right there with you, so I can understand exactly what's going on in these moments?

LIZ: Whenever I feel a headache coming on, I get scared, and I wonder if it's back.

THERAPIST: And the sense of being back in the recovery room, waking up? That comes up, too?

LIZ: Definitely. It was awful! Something went wrong. They didn't tell me, or I didn't hear, what it was going to be like. I had this thin wire running up my spine and fluid emptying out of my brain. When I woke up after the surgery, I must have moved or something, because the pain was just searing. I have never felt anything like that in my life. I mean, delivering a baby is easy compared to this. And I didn't know what was happening. Nobody was there. I panicked. I mean there's a wire up my spine, and I can't move without this searing pain running all the way up to my brain, where they did the surgery. Then, I started to vomit blood. I kept panicking, until they came, gave me some more medicine, and I guess I was out again.

THERAPIST: So now, especially when you get a headache, or a pain in your head or neck, all those pictures and emotions come back?

LIZ: Absolutely! I don't just *see* all this, I *feel* it. I can taste the blood coming up again in those moments. And I can't turn them off! That's the worst part. They'll start when I'm practicing with my band or when I'm at a birthday party with my son. Totally unpredictable. And I think I must be going crazy.

Her PTSD vicious cycle appears in Figure 7.4.

Notice that the traumatic memories are multi-sensory: they are not simply conscious thoughts but involve vivid imagery, body sensations, and even taste sensations. They sometimes spontaneously intruded into awareness. At other times,

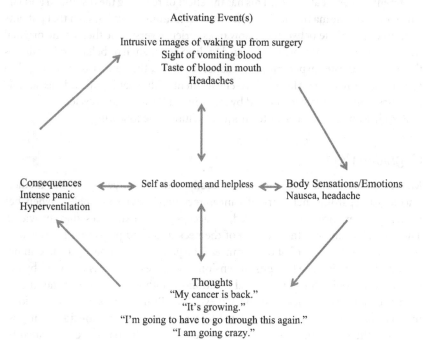

Activating Event(s)

Intrusive images of waking up from surgery
Sight of vomiting blood
Taste of blood in mouth
Headaches

Consequences
Intense panic
Hyperventilation

Self as doomed and helpless

Body Sensations/Emotions
Nausea, headache

Thoughts
"My cancer is back."
"It's growing."
"I'm going to have to go through this again."
"I am going crazy."

FIGURE 7.4 Vicious Cycle: Liz Romano

they appeared to occur when Liz noticed that she had a headache. Eliciting this material created the opportunity for the therapist to provide psychoeducation about memory and re-living in post-traumatic stress. The therapist drew the PTSD cycle, which Mrs. Romano said accurately captured her experiences. Her experiences were normalized in the context of what for anyone would have been an utterly horrifying event: the pain, the sight of tubes and wires in her body, the immobility, the helplessness, and the vomiting of blood constituted a trauma from which Liz could not escape. On top of this, she recently began to believe that her own mind was turning against her when she could not turn off the disturbing imagery and body sensations at will. Believability ratings for her thoughts suggested that during re-living experiences, she believed with about an 8/10 certainty that she was either going crazy or was experiencing a return of her cancer. She experienced self as doomed and helpless at these times.

Ehlers and Clark (2000) described a framework for understanding and intervening in PTSD, as did Hayes, Strosahl, & Wilson (2012). Treatment with Liz Romano involved helping her create a more functional and workable understanding of her experiences. This occurred through psychoeducation about PTSD and by searching for hot spots in her narrative as she worked through the PTSD vicious cycle with the therapist. These cognitive hot spots involve areas in which idiosyncratic and catastrophic meaning is assigned to experiences of a prior trauma. Linking hot spots of the trauma with new information that updates their meaning is also a part of the treatment (Ehlers et al., 2010). This has the effect of reducing the disjointed and jarring nature of trauma memories. Discrimination training occurs, such that patients learn to differentiate between the now of experience versus the then of the original trauma. Patients, finally, are encouraged to drop any mental or behavioral strategies that serve to bolster experiential avoidance. And last, the patient is encouraged to reclaim his or her life by fostering re-engagement with meaningful and pleasurable activities, which have been affected by entry into a PTSD vicious cycle.

For Liz Romano, treatment techniques included the following.

Cognitive Work

Mrs. Romano had already consulted directly with her surgeon and her medical oncologist regarding her fears of cancer recurrence but was unable, when her re-living experiences were triggered, to accept the reassurances they provided. The therapist explored the location of the neck and head pains that Liz was now interpreting as "evidence" of brain cancer. The pains were primarily located in her neck and frontalis muscle, signs of tension headaches. This was affirmed by her medical oncologist. Since the actual location of both the cancer and the intense pain after surgery was near the affected eye, Mrs. Romano was open to considering that her muscle pain was unrelated to cancer. Instead, she considered it possible that the neck pain was related to muscle tension headaches, exacerbated by her stress response. To test this further, she agreed to try a gentle massage of her neck, either self-administered or given by her husband, when she noticed this pain.

Responsiveness to brief massage provided further disconfirmation of the belief that she was experiencing a recurrence of brain cancer. Also, the current and past locations of the pain were different and indicated that the pain was benign: the cancer pain had initially been adjacent to the affected eye, not the back of the neck. The pain of the shunt tube, also, had been positioned differently.

Creating a Present Moment Focus

Present moment exercises were practiced in session, including guided imagery and the 3-minute breathing exercise (Segal et al., 2013), with care taken to deliver these in a manner that did not promote avoidance, but rather the ability to observe experience during a moment-to-pause. As noted before, present moment exercises involve a compassionate, non-judgmental awareness of experience. It is not about relaxation, feeling good, or chasing away bad feelings. It is about developing and maintaining an open, accepting posture toward internal and outer experience.

Perspective-Taking Skills to Create Self-Processes for Cultivating Metacognitive Awareness

A central feature of perspective-taking skills is the ability to promote new stances toward experience. Hayes has described these skills as forming the early core of ACT, which he notes emerged from his own struggles to deal with panic disorder (Hayes, 2016). The use of what Relational Frame Theory describes as deictic frames (Hayes et al., 2001; Villatte et al., 2016) is central in this process, as it is in Ehlers and Clark (2000) and Ehlers et al. (2010). For purposes of this case, we are interested in promoting the experience of me-here-now noticing me-there-then. To simplify this, the task in working with Liz Romano was to help her cultivate the ability to allow the images and sensations of her surgical experience to emerge into awareness, from a place of curiosity and compassion, while noticing and observing those experiences safely, *as events that occurred in the past*. Part of what makes re-living experiences so terrifying in PTSD is their inexplicable intrusiveness into the present moment. The patient lacked a narrative framework for making sense of these experiences, which psychoeducation and other facets of treatment restore (Ehlers & Clark, 2000). Also, and perhaps equally frightening, the patient is left with the sense that the memories and sensations are happening *now*, such that they are not experienced necessarily as memories, but as current moment experiences. This ability to achieve some distance and perspective also helps create a different narrative understanding of the experience, allowing it be present without reacting as though an actual emergency is occurring.

The steps taken are as follows:

1.   Creating a moment-to-pause, mindfully;
2.   Using guided imagery to bring attention to five-senses experiences;

3. Fostering awareness of a self, an observer who is present and noticing five-senses experiences;
4. Noticing the self who has been present in past experiences;
5. Allowing that observing self to be present as suffering and pain emerge into awareness, from a place of caring and compassion and curiosity toward that suffering;
6. Seeing past suffering as past suffering, showing up in the moment;
7. Allowing it to be, without engaging in avoidance behaviors or cognitions;
8. Returning awareness to present moment experiences.

A condensed example of this exercise with Liz Romano might look like this:

THERAPIST: Liz, let's take a moment to again sink into this moment, just to be here, now. Almost like setting down roots, like a big oak tree, right here, now, into this moment. We have nowhere we have to be and nothing else we need to be doing in just this moment. Breathing in, this moment. Breathing out, just this moment . . . now from this place, let's notice the sounds in the room . . . let's shift our awareness to include the sensations in the body . . . the thoughts and images that come up . . . just noticing . . . just allowing awareness to take in what comes up through the five senses, and through our own thoughts and emotions and body sensations. Just awareness . . . now I would ask that you allow into awareness the things that scare you, the images we have talked about, the sensations . . . and I would ask, can you notice all of that from here, now, looking at it with the curiosity and compassion of a long ago time that hurt you? You, here, now . . . just watching . . . just noticing . . . noticing those experiences as they were then . . . and seeing how they can show up now, as memories that feel alive, but from a place of curiosity and compassion . . . compassion to yourself, as you were then in that room, waking up from surgery, not knowing what was happening, and so understandably frightened and in pain. Now, coming back into the room, just noticing body sensations as body sensations . . . memories as memories . . . thoughts and emotions as thoughts and emotions . . . the sounds in the room . . . knowing that this is you, here, now, having memories, or body sensations, emotions, and thoughts, as they are now . . . and whenever you are ready, we'll come back to the room and just talk a bit.

This exercise clearly needs to be done with great tact and clinical sensitivity. It can promote emotion dysregulation otherwise. At the fist whiff of distress, the clinician must assess the patient's ability and willingness, and be prepared to back away if need be, and to more slowly approach the core fears, including the cognitions, body sensations, emotions, and imagery of which they are composed. But for Liz Romano, who was easily able to establish a trusting therapy relationship, and who was motivated, and had considerable adaptive strengths, the exercise was helpful. She became more able to allow in experiences from the past, for what they were: experiences from the past that her mind continued to work over. They needn't have a claim on her life today. It is simultaneously an exposure exercise, an acceptance and present moment exercise, and a perspective-taking exercise. Done in ways that are consistent with available science and theories of PTSD, exercises of this sort can help patients achieve metacognitive awareness of the vicious cycle as well as Theory 2, an alternative narrative that is both more potentially accurate and more functionally useful.

Life Engagement Strategies

ACT emphasizes values and commitment work, not just a focus on changing one's relationship to internal experience. Ehlers et al. (2010) emphasized "reclaiming your life," not just cognitive restructuring. Consistent with our focus on helping people engage with important life contexts and sources of support and meaning, therapy with Liz Romano involved helping her connect more fully with areas of life that mattered to her. Here is what she wrote on a 3 × 5 index card, to take with her:

How to Break Out of This Vicious Cycle

1. Remember: these experiences are memories, not things happening to me now.
2. Let the memories, body sensations, and emotions sit there; they will take care of themselves without my having to do anything to get rid of them.
3. Take my life back: movies, sports, phone calls to friends, work, time with my husband.
4. Carry on: it's a new day, and I have my life back.

Chapter Summary

Anxiety disorders are the most commonly occurring psychological problems in the general population. And they are, along with depression, the most common clinical problems among cancer patients. This chapter reviewed CBT formulations for conceptualizing anxiety disorders, using the anxiety equation. Then, we described maintaining factors for anxiety problems, including cognitive, emotional, and behavioral maintainers. Applications of the principles that guide this book were made in describing the therapy relationship, providing psychoeducational interventions, and for dealing with both the content and process of anxious cognition. Case examples and sample transcripts were provided to show practical strategies for helping anxious cancer patients, including those presenting with features of PTSD, medical phobias, and panic as well as adjustment difficulties.

Key Points

1. The anxiety equation involves the balance between threat estimates and one's capacity to manage, and be helped to manage, threat.

2. Case formulations for anxiety include the use of Guided Discovery to reveal vicious cycles and to create treatment plans that help free patients from anxious vicious cycles.

3. Anxiety is normalized in the context of the evolutionarily adaptive function of fear.

4. Threat estimation by cancer patients is matched against perceived status by the medical teams.

5. Hidden meanings behind cancer-related anxiety can reveal not only cognitive biases but also areas in which problem-solving strategies might be brought to bear on dealing with the grain of truth in feared situations.

6. Worry, including normal and pathological forms, was identified.

7. Clinical strategies to identify and disrupt patterns of chronic worry and anxious arousal were described.

8. Tolerance of uncertainty as well as emotion regulation and distress tolerance strategies are important in working with cancer patients.

9. Strategies to help patients not only alter their relationship to anxious internal content were advanced but also focus on engagement in meaningful activities in life were described.

Eight
Putting a Floor Under the Distressed Patient
Very Brief Therapy with Cancer Patients

Patients in cancer centers are often referred in states of high distress, with limited time or energy for engagement in extensive therapy. While the spectrum of cognitive behavior therapies is often considered to be brief, randomized controlled trials for depression and anxiety disorders often require 12 to 20 sessions. Treatment for long-standing adaptive difficulties, such as borderline personality disorder, may require many months, or years. This stands in contrast to the fact that most people seeking therapy in community settings neither want nor remain in therapy for more than four to six sessions (Olfson et al., 2009; Strosahl et al., 2012). In fact, people are at times capable of making meaningful, clinically significant changes, in a short time, whether or not they continue to meet criteria for *DSM* disorders. And, in CBT for depression and anxiety, patient gains can be sudden and significant (Aderka et al., 2012), often before the presumed mechanisms of treatment have had a chance to be invoked. This leads to the conclusions that our assumptions about therapy duration may be out of touch with what many people seeking help actually want and need from a therapy encounter. In addition, the actual mechanisms of change are not as well understood as we might wish, despite our efforts to create theoretically coherent and empirically supported models. Since people can experience enduring benefits from very brief therapy, we need to think through how to help people get the most from therapy encounters that may last at most a few sessions, without sacrificing the commitment to science and sound theory that is a bedrock of the CBT movement.

Brief psychotherapy models abound (Watzlawick et al., 1974; Gustafson, 1986; 1992; 2005; deShazar, 1988; Epston & White, 1990; Watzlawick, 1993; Budman & Gurman, 2002; Levenson, 2010) including single-session therapy (Talmon, 1990;

Hoyt & Talmon, 2014). For a useful and aptly brief overview of the brief therapy movement and its empirical status, the reader is referred to Strosahl et al. (2012). Adaptations of brief therapy for medical patients (Rosenberg & McDaniel, 2014), including brief CBT for cancer patients, exist (Levin & Applebaum, 2012), owing to the recognition that patients, their families, and their medical teams may have substantial needs but limited time.

Therapy conducted in the hurly burly of a busy cancer clinic, therefore, often involves a single consultation and frequently involves fewer than the four to six sessions that commonly take place in community treatment settings. Therapy must therefore be focused, purposeful, and honed. As an example, time is at a premium for newly diagnosed patients, adjusting to the shock of a cancer diagnosis and the need to mobilize their resources to enter and cope with the rigors of treatment. Even for patients who are deep in long-term survivorship, time may be very limited for psychotherapy: having spent a great deal of time in the cancer center, even years earlier, they may want to get on with life, and have very limited contact with their care team. It is, therefore, important to anticipate brevity when encountering each new patient, and to treat every session, from the first, as a chance to make a difference, now. If the encounter ends up involving a longer time frame, we have set the stage for purposeful treatment, right from the first session.

The mission of very brief therapy is varied. Often, we are asked to help turn around a psychologically deteriorating situation. With highly distressed patients, we must work to provide a floor beneath the distressed person, a metaphor which is useful to impart to the patient that our mission is to help stabilize what might otherwise feel like a free-fall through space. Our primary mission in some cases is to stabilize a patient whose psychological resources are deteriorating. In many other cases, single or brief consultations help patients focus on meeting the adaptive challenges required of them as they face their illness, their treatment, or emerging challenges that may arise later. The organizing principles outlined in Chapter 2 are applicable for very brief interventions with cancer patients. If the treatment protocols in CBT are written for 12–20 session encounters, then we need to find ways to scale down the treatment when fewer sessions are all we have. The brief CBT therapist needs to be focused on the art of the possible, realizing that small steps taken purposefully can reverberate in big and unanticipated ways in the patient's life. We do not have to think in terms of fully resolving depressive episodes or anxiety disorders in order to provide adequate help when time is limited. The objective may be to shore up coping abilities, to help engage people in their care and in life, trusting that they have the wisdom and inner resources to find a path in that life. We can enter each encounter with the awareness that it is possible to make something good happen, right then in session, today. Our work is geared toward creating a rapid formulation, and helping the person create a lifeline into new possibilities. Kirk Strosahl, a co-creator of ACT, likened the work to holding a door open, through which a single step can lead to a new life (Strosahl et al., 2012). It becomes the responsibility of the patient to take that step; it is the therapist's job to help find and hold open the door. James Gustafson, at the University of Wisconsin's Brief Therapy Clinic has observed that he "gives the responsibility back to the patient for what is necessary to get out of the final despair. I leave it to him, and not to me, and thus I am cheerful" (Gustafson, 2005, p. 55).

We can hold the door open via the following:

1. Aim to put a floor under the distressed patient in the first session;
2. Validate the logic of distress;
3. Trust the patient's inner wisdom to be an ally;
4. Mobilize the patient's resources;
5. Rapidly identify key problems and maintaining factors;
6. Think small, but expect results;
7. Create a single focus for therapy;
8. Create a specific action plan by the end of the first session.

What to Know about the Patient Before the First Visit

Collaboration between the therapist and the oncology team is optimal, especially in very brief treatment encounters. Given the structure and time demands of many clinics, time for collaboration can be very limited. The Affordable Care Act, with its emphasis on integration, via medical homes, will likely propel the system toward a more effective inclusion of behavioral health into the care team. For now, it is helpful to begin with a sense of the referring team's concerns. And it is important for the behavioral health consultant to maintain a pipeline of communication with the oncology team(s) in treatment and follow-up. If the patient is directly seeking a consultation, without a referral, it is wise to have the patient complete the ESAS-R, pinpointing global concerns, and the domains of those concerns. If depression and/or anxiety is prominent, a PHQ-9 and a GAD-7 is advised, prior to the first visit. If the therapist has the chance to do a quick review of the record, prior to the first visit, he or she can get a sense of the patient's cancer, the phase of treatment or survivorship of the patient, and perhaps a sense of the team and patient's concerns. An e-mail, a quick visit to key members of the oncology team, or a phone call may provide the best source of information about the reasons for the first visit to the behavioral health professional.

Creating a Treatment Relationship in the Initial Session

The opening moves described in the last chapter are intended to rapidly create an effective treatment relationship, beginning in the first session, and allowing for the possibility that the first session may be the only opportunity to help someone. Joining strategies, Guided Discovery and Socratic Questioning, and validation strategies all are used in the first encounter. By tuning in to the patient's affect, body language, capacity for eye contact, and the patient's narrative, the therapist selects entry points for engagement from among the strategies used in the opening moves. A patient who appears tense and uncertain about seeing a behavioral health professional, and who may have never talked with a psychologist or social worker before, may need a slightly more prolonged period of joining. Then, GD/SQ might be employed, to clarify their expectations about the meeting, or their understanding of the reasons for the referral, and their understanding of the nature of their cancer. Validation strategies dovetail with GD/SQ as a means of creating a trusting, collaborative environment. On the other hand, the patient who comes in with clarity about what he or she wants help with, and who begins talking about key problems and challenges he or she faces, can be engaged with perhaps a minimum of joining efforts. A few key questions guide our inquiry in an initial session:

1. Does the patient know the reason for the referral? Did they request to see the behavioral health team, or did a member of the oncology team refer them? What were they told, and by whom?
2. What is their understanding of their disease?
3. How do they experience their relationship to the medical team that is caring for them?
4. What are they key problems, as they see it, and how are those problems showing up in their daily life?
5. What strategies have they tried to manage those key problems, and with whose help?
6. Is the patient's distress tolerance and emotion regulation being eroded by sleep problems, pain, suicidal ideation, and intense stress arousal?

We must try to make at least a provisional formulation by the end of the first session. This will include not only mobilizing resources for a psychotherapeutic strategy, but referral for medication therapy, as indicated.

Tuning in to the Patient's Stance Toward Cancer

Moorey and Greer (2012) focused on the patient's adjustment style which, to review, include fighting spirit, denial, fatalism, helplessness/hopelessness, and anxious preoccupation. Nezu et al. (2007; 2012) also described the range of problem orientations that can impede or enhance the ability to effectively cope with cancer's challenges. These include an impulsive, avoidant, or rational problem-solving style. Effective brief therapy for cancer requires the therapist to attune rapidly to the patient's adjustment and problem-solving stance, via attunement to his or her use of language, metaphor, and body language. Our efforts may initially involve helping to kindle or re-access a more effective problem-solving style, as a precursor to engagement in more active coping strategies.

Chapter 2 highlighted the idea that humans process information in multiple modes, one of which is through the more rational, explicitly verbal mode. The other is a more implicit mode, which is often encoded in imagery and metaphor. We want to help normalize and frame problems using whichever mode is most effective for any given patient. Since implicit encoding of meaning appears to be the more rapid and emotionally laden mode (Teasdale, 1999; Kahneman, 2011), the use of imagery and metaphor is worth honing (Stott et al., 2010; Hackmann et al., 2011; Hayes, Strosahl, & Wilson, 2012; Stoddard & Afari, 2014).

One metaphor that can help normalize and validate patient distress, reframe self in relation to problems, and set the stage for effective problem-solving is *The Juggler Metaphor*. The therapist invites the patient to consider how easily one can juggle a single ball, tossing it up in the air all day, if need be, and catching it when it drops. If a second ball is added, it may be achievable, but more difficult. Then a third. Then a fourth. Then a fifth, by which time the therapist and the patient may be in agreement that there is a limit to the number of balls that one can juggle. The therapist explains that such factors as history, temperament, and practice determine how many balls, or how many complex items in life, one can juggle. For anyone, a limit is reached, beyond which one's coping reserves become frayed. Even the most skilled of jugglers will reach the point at which everything asked by life cannot be juggled effectively. By going through the daily list of activities or duties in the patient's life, and by adding the demands and limitations imposed by cancer and cancer therapies, the patient can begin to recognize that even the most skilled of jugglers has a limit. It can be a relief to simply recognize that cancer provides a valid reason to re-think daily priorities, to ask for help when needed, to reduce work hours where possible, to delegate responsibilities where feasible, and to accept limitations, even temporarily. The image of balls or bowling pins in the air can serve to cue the creation of a problem list which, in turn, lends itself to a more problem-solving focus, as indicated. Here is a brief therapy transcript, demonstrating the use of the metaphor with a patient.

PATIENT: I can't think straight. I'm so worried all the time and so upset, I don't know where to start. The kids have to carry on; they have school and routines and soccer practice. My spouse needs my support. The bills have to get paid. Work has to get done at the office. My mom still needs me to get groceries to her every week. I'm on the board of directors at my church. And now this. Cancer. Chemotherapy. And maybe surgery after that, if the chemo shrinks the tumor enough. I can't think straight and I can't sleep any more.

THERAPIST: What if what you're going through is like juggling? Too many balls in the air, and we can't keep them all going.

PATIENT: What do you mean?

THERAPIST: Well, it might be like this (Taking a small colored foam ball from the desk drawer, and holding it in hand, beginning to toss it aloft and catch it). I could probably keep this going for a long time. How about you?

PATIENT: All day, if I had to.

THERAPIST: Me too. Now what if I take another one out? (Gets a second colored foam ball and tosses it aloft, catching it while the other one is tossed in the air) I can do this for a while, but it's harder. (Sets balls aside) Suppose I had a third? A fourth? A fifth one?

PATIENT: Down they go.

THERAPIST: Yes. Down they go. For you, too?

PATIENT: Most definitely. I think I see where this is going.

THERAPIST: We all reach a point where the number of things that life throws at us exceeds our comfort zone for coping. It's the way life works. Now let's take a look at what you said a few minutes ago. It seems to me that you've been a very good juggler your whole life, if you can juggle kids, career, finances, being married, looking after mom, and being on boards. That's a lot of successful juggling.

PATIENT: I hadn't looked at it like that. It's just what I do. It's my life.

THERAPIST: Yes, it's your life, and you seem pretty good at it. But then this thing extra new thing came along, called cancer. Out of the blue. And with it, chemotherapy. Then surgery. Then waiting to see what's next. What's that like to juggle all that, on top of everything else in your life?

PATIENT: It's overwhelming.

Creating a Problem List in Very Brief Therapy

In a sense, behavioral health clinicians working in a cancer center don't have to fish for a problem list facing their patients. Cancer itself creates a problem list. However, we don't know how cancer is experienced or elaborated by our patients, without using GD/SQ to find out. And we don't know how cancer is experienced by their social support systems or what roadblocks to effective coping may be in the patient's path. It's wise to get a sense of these in the first session. Key problems in very brief therapy often include one or more of the following:

1. The patient needs emotional support and validation, which for one reason or another is not available or is not being accessed in the patient's daily life.
2. The patient needs to create a sense of meaning and order to a disrupted sense of self and world.
3. Coping strategies that worked in the past do not work now.
4. Distress tolerance is being eroded in ways that limit effective problem solving.
5. Cancer-related pain and fatigue may be creating vulnerabilities to depression and anxiety and must be targeted for both change and acceptance work.

Any one or any combination may be present. We engage the patient in a collaborative process to:

1. Identify the vicious cycle in which they are currently stuck;
2. Create a new pattern that allows for more effective problem management;
3. Create interventions that foster taking first steps toward a new pattern, or re-engagement with adaptive patterns that have worked in the past.

Let's turn to clinical examples.

Using Patient Metaphors to Create a Rapid Formulation for Problem Solving

Even prior to generating the data necessary for a more thorough case formulation, it is possible, at times necessary, to create a mini-formulation and a shared treatment agreement in the first session of therapy. Metaphor, using the patient's language, can provide a means of setting an initial agreement about problem areas, giving the patient the sense that his or her suffering is understood and that he or she will have an ally in treatment.

The Case of the Woman Who Lost Her Voice

A 36-year-old married mother of two children is referred through palliative care, where she is seen for pain management following surgical removal 9 months ago of her larynx for a Stage III cancer. While the surgery was deemed successful, in terms of cancer removal, she now speaks with the aid of an electrical device placed against her throat. This leaves her with a mechanical, robotic speech pattern, of which she is ashamed. In the first session, when asked not just what she understood to be the team's reason for referral, she said: "I'm lost. I feel like I've turned into a ghost. Nobody notices me anymore."

Albert Camus (1955) wrote, "to come back to life, we need grace, a homeland, or to forget ourselves" (p. 165). We can hypothesize that this patient feels homeless and adrift, without interpersonal support or resources. The image of being a ghost, invisible and lost, is stunningly powerful and evocative. Following up on that imagery, the therapist included the idea of helping the patient becoming audible, being heard. In addition, the imagery of being lost prompted the therapist to use another metaphor of a map: "What if we could create a map together, one in which you can find a path back to people, and to being heard?" Neither the therapist nor the patient needs to know the steps at this point. These will need to be explored in detail.

In fact, the therapist and the patient identified her refusal to talk as a problem. Filled with shame at the sound of her robotic voice, she was left feeling like an unheard ghost by her family. The therapist encouraged the patient to create a map, literally writing out a map that would bring her home to her family. She had avoided speaking, and had instead opted for writing notes to her family until, by her own recognition, they were becoming weary from reading her handwritten notes. In helping the patient take the perspectives of her husband and children, she was able to risk using the electronic device to speak. In a second session, she reported that the family, especially her children, were responsive. She felt less like a ghost, and more like someone who had rediscovered her homeland.

Emotional Support and Validation: The Elderly Man Who Read Atul Gawande

Sometimes, the patient's coping strategies and juggling abilities are not only good but also may be underappreciated by others. Validating the patient, including his or her coping strategies, can be pivotal in very brief therapy.

An example:

An oncologist referred 80-year old Herb Shayler for assessment of depression. Mr. Shayler has a new recurrence of advanced prostate cancer and had been treated in the past with steroids, to manage inflammation associated with chemotherapies. The steroids induced the only depressive episode of Mr. Shayler's life, and he is loath to endure another round of steroids, even if the chemotherapy offers a greater promise of extending life than the alternative medicine. The oncologist would like to encourage Mr. Shayler to consider the medication that would require the steroids and have the behavioral health team help him cope with depression, should it recur.

The initial meeting involved the oncologist, an oncology fellow, the psychologist, Mr. Shayler, and Mr. Shayler's daughter, who accompanies him to the cancer center each time. Mr. Shayler sat with his arms crossed and was openly wary about having a psychologist included in the meeting. He indicated that he believed that the team wanted him to take the chemotherapy option that would require steroids, but that he would not do so just on their recommendation. He would make up his own mind. He expressed concern that the team believed that he is not making a rational choice. After learning the two available options, the best offering no more than perhaps another 18 months of life, he stated that he would think about the options. He turned to the psychologist and said, "People like you probably think I ought to do anything to extend my life, even for a little longer. But maybe quality matters more than length." He was surprised when the psychologist agreed that life extension, at all costs, is not necessarily wise. In addition, the psychologist explored the past depressive episode, which was severe, and which robbed Mr. Shayler of his very sense of self. He was a fiercely independent and determined man, accustomed to being busy, engaged socially, and active in home repair and helping others. The prior depression made all of those cherished domains of life impossible. He had no intention to revisit this experience, even if the treatment might extend life by a matter of months. Mr. Shayler agreed to give the matter a bit of reflection, perhaps as a nod to the team's insistence, and he agreed reluctantly to meet with the psychologist when he returned in two weeks.

In the follow-up meeting, Mr. Shayler's daughter encouraged her father to meet alone with the psychologist, while she waited in the lobby. Mr. Shayler expressed concerns that the psychologist might think that he was depressed and unable to make a competent decision to choose an option that was less likely to extend life, but more likely to give him a good quality of life at the end. He strongly denied that he was suicidal or depressed. In fact, he said he would very much like to live longer, but not at any cost. He filled out the PHQ-9, which reveals no evidence of depression and was consistent not only with the clinical interviews but also with his daughter's report.

HERB: I've thought about this. I don't want to take the chemotherapy I took it last time. It ruined my quality of life. Do you think that we ought to live longer, no matter what? I don't. I read a book since I last talked with you, *Being Mortal*, by Atul Gawande.

THERAPIST: I know the book. I read it, too. Tell me what came to your mind from that.

             (Atul Gawande is a neurologist and writer whose book is a profound medical and ethical meditation on end-of-life issues, with an element of a memoir included, as Gawande reflects on his own father's end-of-life struggles. Gawande asks readers to consider when it is wise to refrain from the medical heroics and invasive treatments that characterize end-of-life care, toward a more accepting and perhaps humane stance toward death and dying)

HERB: He says what I'm saying. When it's time, it's time. Don't prolong the inevitable, especially when it just causes suffering. I'm not at all afraid to die. I have no fear. And if my wife were here, she'd tell me to do just what I am going to do. I want to take the medicine that has the least likelihood of extending my life, but that doesn't have the effect on me that the other one had. If it works, great, I'll have more time. If not, I'm ready to go. (Patient makes eye contact with the therapist, with his jaw set in a determined, but defensive look)

THERAPIST: I think you're a wise man. And a strong one. I'm delighted you read that book. Tell me more about how it resonated with you.

We then talked about the ideas in the book, and Mr. Shayler was pleased to know that I did not think depression was clouding his judgment, and that I wasn't going to try to push him toward taking the medicines that might extend life, even for a few months longer, but possibly put him back into a crushing depression.

For the first time, Mr. Shayler visibly relaxed, smiled, and extended a hand to shake my hand. "Thank you," he said.

When I had the oncology fellow come in, I asked him if he had read *Being Mortal*. He had not. I explained my findings and recommendations to the resident, and I left Mr. Shayler to give him a brief book review, before the two discussed his chemotherapy choice. I went to the lobby for Mr. Shayler's daughter and talked with her on the way back to the consultation room, where she would join her father. She believed he was wise, capable, and in full command of his decision-making capacity, and that he wanted to go out as he lived, a man in charge of his own destiny.

Two months later, as I went into the clinic lobby for another patient, Mr. Shayler and I saw one another. He was in the clinic again with his daughter, for an oncology follow-up. He smiled, extended his hand, and said, "I haven't read any new books lately." I said, "You read the one that counted."

Downsizing Cancer by Using a Spatial Metaphor and Problem-Solving Strategies

We have seen how cancer can come to dominate a person's life in a way that literally crowds out other, more important domains of functioning. Depressive withdrawal, isolation, and a sense that one has no options, compresses the patient's life, forming what Strosahl and Robinson (2008) referred to as "depression compression." Yet sometimes depression compression can be reversed rapidly, depending upon the patient, the timing of the therapy encounter, and the application of the right model. The following case demonstrates the use of a spatial metaphor to help set the stage for re-engagement in life, followed by specific behavioral steps leading to re-engagement.

Rebecca Whitaker was a 37-year-old formerly successful career woman, married, with three young children. Two years after initial diagnosis with a rare form of cancer, her life had become shrunken by depressive problems and preoccupation with cancer. Her physical appearance had been altered by surgery and her energy diminished by chemotherapy. She worried about her competency and her appearance. The longer she was out of the work force, the greater her worries about no longer being competent or marketable. This further eroded her willingness and ability to leave home, other than to do basic shopping and child care activities.

Her stated problem was that she was "overwhelmed," which is itself a metaphor. The therapist asked, "If this room were the size of your life, how much space would cancer be taking up?" The patient readily stated that three quarters of the room was taken over by cancer. Drawing a circle on a new sheet of paper, using a pie chart technique from Cognitive Therapy, the patient filled in the 75% that represented the space taken up by her cancer. The remaining areas were divided into other life domains: children, self, spouse, work, church, exercise, finances, recreation, and friends. Now, a second pie chart was drawn on a new sheet of paper. The patient was asked to fill it in according to how much space each area deserved. In this case, cancer took up only 25% of the pie, reversing the size of cancer in her current life. The therapist referred to the sheet in which cancer took up only 25% of the patient's life, rather than 75%.

THERAPIST: What if we could begin to find some ways to give cancer the space it deserves, and no more? Twenty-five percent, right? That'd give you a lot more space for other things that matter to you.

REBECCA: I'd like to have the other areas get bigger. I'd like to find some new work, even though I worry about what I look like. And my friends have given up on me, because I keep saying "no" to them when they call me to get together.

THERAPIST: So suppose our work involved getting these parts of the pie a little bigger, and give cancer a smaller place in your life?

REBECCA: I'd like to do that.

The patient's willingness to engage suggested that she was perhaps at a turning point, in the sense that she might benefit from therapy, perhaps rapidly. Using behavioral activation and problem-solving strategies, she mapped a course that involved contacting friends and using makeup to see if she might feel better about her appearance. These seemingly small steps, chosen by the patient and not the therapist, did, in fact, lead to an upward spiral that subsequently resulted in a career move and a more engaged life.

Using Interpersonal Problem-Solving Skills: The Case of the Worried Woman in the Chemotherapy Suite

Celia Parker was 45, married, and had three children. She presented with a metastatic colon cancer and a recently discovered new tumor growth. She was having chemotherapy, which would be followed by surgery. The oncologist referred her because he noticed that Celia was becoming more fearful and worried than he'd seen her before. Facing chemotherapy and another surgery, both of which she had done in prior episodes of cancer care, she was now finding it difficult to cope.

In the first session, in the chemo suite, Celia appeared fretful, worried, and tearful. The therapist's first hypothesis was that she was afraid not only of surgery but also of the possibility that this would be the recurrence that kills her. In fact, Celia's primary concern was the possibility of family conflict erupting when her parents came to town during her surgery, to "support" her. She described a state of "guerrilla war" between her husband, her oldest son, and her parents, especially her mother. Celia experienced the recurrent visual image that while she was under the anesthetic, and recovering from her surgery, "all hell will break loose" in her family. She was upset at the possibility, especially because "I won't be there to manage everyone. I'll be asleep."

The first session involved generating information related to her biggest concern for the moment, how her family would behave toward one another while she was in surgery. The second session involved planning interventions. A subsequent follow-up occurred months later.

Key problems included:

1. Family conflict, which the patient feared would erupt in her absence during surgery.

Maintaining factors included:

1. Beliefs to the effect that "left to their own devices, my family will blow up during my surgery, and it will never be fixed afterwards" and "only I can prevent my mother, my husband, and oldest son from causing a permanent blowup."
2. Long-standing helplessness in the face of her mother's behavior, described as "overpowering and out of control."
3. Beliefs that her husband was incapable of managing himself effectively during her surgery, contrary to available evidence to the contrary.
4. A history of avoidant coping in the face of interpersonal conflict, with efforts to placate others, rather than actively solve interpersonal problems in other, more flexible, ways.

The therapist also helped the patient deal with her fears of an impending family rupture.

THERAPIST: So what do you think the chances are that there'll be a permanent blowup, so that when you wake up from surgery, nobody's going to be speaking to one another?

CELIA: I don't know. My husband is protective of me, and he doesn't really like my mother. He puts up with her. That's about all. But my mom can't be reasoned with, and my dad never takes her on.

THERAPIST: So you have this idea that you're the only person who can keep these warring parties from going to war with one another?

CELIA: That's kind of been my job. But it's pretty hard to do that job when I'm anesthetized.

THERAPIST: I'm thinking if there were a way to be a mediator while unconscious, you'd be the one to do it.

CELIA: (Laughs) It's an impossible situation for me I guess.

THERAPIST: If you talked with your husband about what you're worried about, what would he say?

CELIA: He'd probably say not to worry. That he'll handle it.

THERAPIST: Well, you've been with him for a lot of years. Do you think he can be counted on to handle it?

CELIA: Probably. But I just don't want to wake up from surgery, with all of them in the room angry. I want to feel peaceful when I wake up.

THERAPIST: OK. So what if we started by seeing what we can do to help you wake up in peace?

CELIA: That would be really, really helpful.

The therapist and the patient used problem-solving strategies to then create a plan that would be most likely to insure a peaceful environment when she emerged from the anesthetic. This involved trusting that her husband would not only keep the peace but also make sure that anyone who might be agitated and distressed would not be in the hospital room when Celia woke up from surgery. She talked directly with her husband, to turn over to him her responsibilities for being the peacekeeper and sheriff. She accepted the possibility that a big blowup might occur while she was in surgery, as long as she could wake up peacefully with at least her husband in the room. That, coupled with distress tolerance and mindfulness skills, formed the three-session therapy prior to Celia's having surgery.

The Case of the Woman Who Needed to Be Held at Night

One of the sources of emotion regulation and soothing, as we have seen, comes from validation by others. Behind that, perhaps, lies the evolutionary core of our need for love, connection, and soothing, embedded not only in our prolonged developmental vulnerabilities when young but also our need for tribal support and inclusion (Gilbert, 2009a; Hayes & Sanford, 2014). Therein may lie not only a reality of human life but also an ally in treatment, connecting people to sources of soothing and support from others. Interpersonal Therapy employs similar strategies (Stuart & Robertson, 2012), and CBT, combining contextual principles, emotion regulation, and distress tolerance skills as well as problem-solving strategies, does the same. Sandra Jameson was a 41-year-old woman, a writer, poet, and professor, who was been diagnosed with breast cancer, and was referred for what her oncologist regarded as a possible depressive or anxiety disorder. In the first of two sessions, she indicated that she had never seen a psychologist before and had not been diagnosed or treated for depression or anxiety problems in the past. The ESAS-R, the PHQ-9, and the GAD-7 showed distress, without clear indications of a serious depressive or anxiety disorder. She stated that since the diagnosis of a Stage I breast cancer, she had been fearful, worried, and alone. She was married and had two young children. She was fearful of burdening her husband, who was struggling with the demands of his busy life, now added to by his wife's cancer. She was especially distressed at night, when it was dark, her husband was asleep, and she was alone in their bed with her fears and worries. Her worries were what Wells (2009) described as Type I worry, essentially normal human worry, involving the fear of cancer, surgery, after effects, success of treatment, and a fear of eventually dying young. It was at night that her fears exploded, and kept her up sometimes until 2:00 a.m., even though she had to get up early to deal with her children and to get to work herself at the university. We, therefore, pegged her night fears as a problem for focus in our first session. It appeared that her beliefs about being a burden, and about intruding on her husband's need for rest, were keeping her from turning to a key source of support and soothing in her moments of greatest need. One potential strategy might have been to ask her to test her beliefs against the evidence, or to do an experiment in which she asked her husband directly. The latter step would involve encouraging her to act opposite to her current strategy of avoidance, which was also maintaining her isolation and fear.

THERAPIST: Who was it who said three a.m. is the dark night of the soul?
SANDRA: F. Scott Fitzgerald.
THERAPIST: What are you doing in those dark hours to try to comfort or calm yourself?
SANDRA: I just lay there, worrying, picturing everything that might go wrong.
THERAPIST: Not much comfort in that, is there?
SANDRA: No. Not much. Sometimes I get up to read, or to watch TV. Or I make some hot chocolate.
THERAPIST: What have you done at other times, when you needed some comfort?
SANDRA: My husband comforts me.
THERAPIST: But not at midnight?
SANDRA: He's sleeping then, and he needs his sleep. I don't want to bother him.

We explored the belief that she would be a bother. This included asking her to say whether she would be bothered, if he were in a similar situation and needed her support. We also did some perspective-taking work, encouraging Sandra to imagine her husband's reaction to her need, if he were to know, and his possible reaction if she were hurting, yet refused to ask him for help. I asked her to imagine what her husband would say if he knew that Sandra was suffering and alone in her "dark night of the soul."

SANDRA: He'd say to wake him up, if I needed to.
THERAPIST: So he would likely not say "Don't bother me; I have a busy life"?
SANDRA: No. I don't really think he'd say that at all. In fact, I'm guessing, now that I think about it, that he'd probably be a little miffed at me if I wrote him off like that.
THERAPIST: I like him already, and I haven't even met him.
SANDRA: He's a sweetie.
THERAPIST: Yeah. It sounds like it. So how might he comfort you if you let him know you were hurting, alone, and scared?
SANDRA: He'd hold me, and maybe not even have to say anything.
THERAPIST: And how would that feel? Let's just take a moment to quietly imagine that you were held, silently.
         (Silence)
SANDRA: (Eyes closed, visualizing and imagining; breathes slowly) I feel more at peace.
THERAPIST: So what might that be saying to you? If that sense of peace is a message, from you to you, what's it saying?

SANDRA: That I need to be held at night, and that my husband would probably not only do it, he'd be hurt and upset if he thought I was suffering and wouldn't ask him for help.

The patient agreed to try this seemingly simple strategy and return for a follow-up visit in another week. She was scheduled for surgery and chemotherapy the following week and agreed to follow up if she ever felt the need for additional therapy. In the meantime, the social support and the physical soothing from her husband at night were sufficient to bring palpable relief to her in her dark night of the soul.

A Word on Medication Therapy

The cases presented all highlight the use of psychological interventions. Many of the strategies used in treating depression and anxiety problems are applicable in dealing with distress in brief therapy: the 3-minute breathing exercise, DBT distress tolerance skills, various self-processes. However, in situations where the patient is falling through the floor of his or her adaptive reserves, and where mindfulness, distress tolerance skills, and problem-solving skills are unlikely to be effectively utilized, it is wise to consider the addition of medication. Similarly, if the patient has a preference for medication over psychotherapy, this is to be honored. When prolonged, intense distress is present, along with pain, sleeplessness, and/or eroding attentional and cognitive resources, we have to halt suffering rapidly. Failing to put a floor beneath the deteriorating patient may result in a psychiatric hospitalization, failure or refusal to adhere to potentially life-saving medical regimens, or frank suicidality. Short-term anxiolytics, sleep agents, and/or SSRIs have a role in dampening intense psychophysiological distress. If patients pass the crisis period and are able to reinvoke prior adaptive abilities, medication can be backed away from. If longer term work is required to help patients, they can be encouraged to re-engage in CBT or consider longer term trials of medication. In these cases, the CBT therapist must work collaboratively with the medical teams to rapidly stabilize highly distressed patients, who are facing immediate and at times frightening medical procedures.

Chapter Summary

This chapter set a rationale for very brief therapy encounters, using an integrative approach to CBT to spark acceptance and change processes. Based on the assumption that patient strengths and resources are an available ally, brief encounters can foster and mobilize those resources, set a course for change, and lead to greater hope and improved problem-solving, sometimes quite rapidly. The brief CBT therapist is encouraged to see the possible in the present moment and to flexibly and creatively employ the organizing principles from Chapter 2, to help foster acceptance and change in the stuck moments that have occasioned the patient's referral to us for help. Examples of both very brief and more extended therapies were provided in Chapters 6 and 7 on the treatment of depression and anxiety problems, respectively.

Key Points

1. Rapidly identify key problems and maintaining factors.
2. Assess for the presence of cancer-related pain and fatigue, which may be creating vulnerabilities for depression, anxiety and other adjustment difficulties.
3. Validate the logic of distress.
4. Mobilize the patient's fighting spirit.
5. Create a single focus for therapy.
6. Very brief therapy deals with the art and science of the possible: think small, but expect results.
7. Trust the patient's inner wisdom to be an ally.
8. Normalize distress in the face of challenges that tax resources.
9. Aim to put a floor under the distressed patient, using the model and medication, as indicated.
10. Tune in to what the patient is not seeing, which may be maintaining his or her problems.
11. Be in problem-solving mode.
12. Create a single step forward by the end of the first session.

Nine
Therapist Self-Care and Self-Practice

"In taking up another's cross, one must sometimes get crushed by the weight."
—Paul Kalanithi (2016)

No reasonable person would suggest that to become a more effective and compassionate medical oncologist, one should take Tamoxifen, a powerful cancer medication. Or expose oneself to full brain radiation therapy. Certainly, to do so would instill empathy for the patient who must endure the side effects of treatment. But it would not only be unwise; it would be an act of madness. Yet psychotherapy is probably best delivered from a place of both personal conviction in its efficacy, and through the personal use of the model, by applying it in one's own life (Padesky, 1996; Bennett-Levy et al., 2015).

CBT has evolved in directions that seem to take us far from its early behavioral and then cognitive roots. Increasingly, CBT, writ large, has moved in the directions outlined in this book. It remains true to its scientific underpinnings and aspirations, with coherent theories based on testable hypotheses, offering an abundance of clinical tool kits that flow from the theories. At the same time, CBT is increasingly concerned with living a purposeful, meaningful, engaged life, a life that matters, even in tough circumstances. Newer CBT models increasingly draw from the world's spiritual, meditative, and contemplative traditions, though casting the techniques in the crucible of a science of psychology. In addition, advances in the neurosciences have helped us understand how certain processes such as mindfulness and acceptance as well as self-processes involving perspective taking and compassion can be activated and represented not only behaviorally and experientially but also in our neurophysiology (Davidson & Begley, 2012;

Singer & Bolz, 2013; Ricard, 2015). Without cultivation of sensible practices, in supportive environments, therapists can fall prey to burnout (Figley, 1995). It is increasingly evident that newer CBT models are not just about our patients but also about us. The self-practice of the principles outlined in this book can deepen not only our effectiveness as clinicians, but also our sense of well-being, and enhance the disciplined use of self, which lies at the heart of our work. Personally, and quite frankly, I had to learn these lessons after a painful experience earlier in my career.

Many years ago, I led a 3-year project, working with families of inner city youth homicide victims. I published about the work, which led to contacts with therapists in Northern Ireland, where I was invited to visit, and where I collaborated in a national conference in Belfast, on working with victims of war trauma. But by then, I had become despondent. I uncharacteristically began to drink too much. I withdrew. I felt helpless and ashamed of my own good life, of the fact that my wife and my children lived good, safe lives, when so many in our society suffer cruel and unfair fates, because of the color of their skin or the accident of birth into one socioeconomic level or another. In sum, I became deeply depressed. One night, at dinner in a restaurant with my wife, I said that I knew I had to take time away from clinical practice. I then withdrew from practice for a full year. We lived off our savings and my wife's income as a teacher. I wrote two books and completed a master's degree in health policy and management during that time. After that, I came back to clinical practice, teaching, and research, determined to learn from the experience of my own burnout and to find a "new path to the waterfall" as the writer/poet Raymond Carver put it. I believe I have. In fact, the principles outlined in this book helped me understand why I fell prey to burnout in the first place and what all of us might do to maintain a high level of engagement and effectiveness for our patients and for the teams with whom we work.

Using Principles of the Book in Self-Care/Self-Practice

A Normalizing View of Human Suffering

The distress from having cancer includes not only facing the possibility of a markedly changed life but also the possible looming threat of death. The healers, too, will experience distress at times, pierced as we can be by the pain and suffering of our patients. How could it be otherwise? Accepting that illness and death are a part of life is at the center of world wisdom traditions. So is the struggle to stave off both. Therapists working with cancer patients need not only the science and clinical skills that CBT models bring forth. We also need strategies to manage and accept the pain evoked within us, and our teams, by being with those who are suffering. We want to find ways to let emotional pain inform and guide us, not blow us off course into burnout and despair.

The Disciplined Use of the Therapist's Self in Fostering the Treatment Relationship

We have seen that a central tool in the delivery of effective CBT for cancer is the person of the therapist. In MBCT, for example, not only is the therapist expected to maintain a mindfulness practice but also it appears that the compassion of the therapist may be a factor in sparking the cultivation of compassion in the patients, even without formally using compassion and lovingkindness meditations (Segal et al., 2013). Recent research on the neurobiology and psychology of compassion suggest that there are significant differences between empathy and compassion, and these differences have important implications for anyone working with people who suffer. Empathy involves the activation of brain circuitries implicated in pain: when our patients hurt, we hurt. The same pain circuitries activated in our patients become activated in the therapist (Singer & Bolz, 2013). This level of pain is highly aversive and contributes to avoidance, depression, helplessness, and burnout. Empathy itself is capable of tanking the therapist, psychophysiologically. In fact, the well-known term "compassion fatigue" might rather be renamed "empathic distress fatigue" (Singer & Bolz, 2013, p. 470). Compassion, on the other hand, activates different brain circuitry. Tania Singer, at the Max Planck Institute for Human Cognitive and Brain Sciences, has found that in states of compassion, the person is deeply aware of the pain of the other, though in a state of caring and equanimity, paired with the intention to alleviate suffering. Matthieu Ricard, a former microbiologist and long-time Buddhist monk, was studied at the Max Planck Institute, and notes that in states of compassion, rather than empathy, he is "activating the warm, loving caring feeling which a mother would activate toward a crying child."

However, compassion is not dependent upon achieving a specific emotional state, in and of itself. Compassion, in contrast, makes room for pain, one's own and that of one's patients, yet remains anchored in acceptance and in the intention to relieve suffering. In fact, it may be evoked best in states of equanimity and emotion regulation. Too much emotion arousal—fear, a wish to flee, anger, sadness—can swamp compassion.

Just as compassion thrives in states of emotion regulation and equanimity, so, too, do humor and creativity thrive in a state of emotion regulation. Therefore, the disciplined use of the therapist's self involves the cultivation of compassion, including self-compassion, emotion regulation, equanimity, humor, and creativity. Therapist compassion is central, and it must be nurtured by the therapist and ideally by the contexts and ecosystems in which the therapist is embedded. The principles that follow will focus on practices that might foster such states and processes.

Spotting Therapy-Derailing and Burnout-Inducing Beliefs

Just as patients can bring therapy-interfering cognitions and behaviors to the table, so, too, can therapists. Behavioral health clinicians are wise to use the tools of

CBT to genuinely assess their own beliefs about themselves and their work (Leahy, 2001). In addition, self-practice/self-reflection can foster not only a deepening of the therapist's skills but also the kind of personal growth that is intertwined with evolving competencies in the model (Bennett-Levy et al., 2015). Learning to spot our own cognitive biases, our own rigid and inflexible rules and assumptions, and our own areas of avoidance, will not only increase our effectiveness but also can spare us suffering. For example, imagine a behavioral health clinician who believes "I cannot stand to see a young mother die," or "I must be able to help any patient who comes to me," or "I can't stand to feel too much sadness," or "I have to feel affection for all my patients." Either one develops a more flexible and metacognitive stance vis-à-vis such beliefs, as well as a more open and accepting stance toward feared emotions, or burnout may ensue. If one can honestly conclude that such flexibility will not be forthcoming, it is better to know that, accept this, and to choose one's clinical focus and caseload accordingly. There is absolutely no shame in knowing one's current limitations and honoring them; they can be revisited at any time. That is one of the benefits of clinical work; it can spark growth when we are ready for it. In my own case, I harbored unrealistic expectations of myself and of my treatment models. I believed that I "should" be able to help the families, including young siblings, mothers, fathers, and grandparents who were devastated by the murder of their family members. When family members lapsed into despair, drug or alcohol abuse, or treatment termination, I believed that I had failed them. You can see where this would lead.

Now take a few moments to reflect on your key beliefs, including mental images, which have some emotional resonance for you. If you are part of a consultation group, or a team in which high trust exists, feel free to ask others how they might characterize your own beliefs and stance toward the work. Write down those hot cognitions when they begin to take shape for you, regarding your own beliefs, rules, and assumptions about therapy:

1. _____
2. _____
3. _____
4. _____
5. _____

See how those might match up with such beliefs as these:

1. I am committed to improving my skills, for the rest of my career, knowing that I am an imperfect healer and will always be.
2. I commit to easing the suffering of my patients to the best of my and their ability to do so.
3. I commit to embarking on a path of acceptance, that pain is an inherent part of a human life, mine included. Pain is not the enemy.

4. I will trust that my patients have vast reserves of strength and wisdom that they can and will bring to bear on dealing with their circumstances. I trust that I also have such reserves of wisdom.

5. I am a catalyst for change, but I am not responsible for making people change. At best, I can open a door. I will trust that my patients will know when to, or if they should, walk through the door to changing their lives.

6. People are not broken, and they do not necessarily need therapy or CBT in order to find a path in life.

The alternative beliefs I offer are not the "right" answers. I don't have right answers. They are some of the ways of looking at this work that I have come up with for myself. I will provide an opportunity for you, later, to generate some potentially new rules and assumptions of your own.

Building Resilient Self-Processes and Ways of Being

An opening move in building resilient self-processes and new ways of being (Bennett-Levy et al., 2015), is through mindfulness. Mindfulness practices foster the capacity to attend to experience, and to stay with experience, regardless of the content of that experience. This, in turn, can help build the muscles of acceptance and compassion. ACT, DBT, and MBCT all foster practices of mindfulness, ranging from experiential exercises in session to more formal periods of seated meditation. While these practices have a spiritual dimension to them, they are initially focused on building attentional processes. Then, we practice staying with experience, including both aversive and pleasant experience, without clinging or pushing such experiences away. The purpose of this is to cultivate the ability to freely choose how to relate to both aversive and pleasant experience, without either pushing it away in a knee-jerk manner, or persisting with it when perhaps letting go is the wise and flexible move.

With flexible, sustained awareness and attention, we strengthen the ability to be with what emerges into awareness, what the Buddhist teacher Pema Chödrön called the ability to "just stay," knowing that we humans have a tendency to flee from pain (Chödrön, 2001). This, in turn, builds the muscle of acceptance. Sitting in session with a young mother, dying of brain cancer, her baby on her knee, is potentially a highly aversive experience for the therapist. Sitting in session with a young adult, similarly facing the delay, if not the derailment, of his dreams in life, due to cancer, can similarly evoke intense pain. Learning to accept that disease is a part of life, which our best science can so far not erase, is a wise and necessary move by the therapist. Compassion for self and others, with the gentle intention of easing the suffering of others, is brought to bear on the clinical encounter.

Compassion training can foster more resilient self-processes in therapists. Mindfulness training fosters metacognitive awareness, or what ACT considers a defused, lightly held experience of internal content, with compassion and acceptance. Yet specific training in cultivating compassion is also warranted. As described earlier, empathy and compassion are not the same processes. To feel another's pain is not enough to insure effective healing or freedom from burnout. Compassion involves an awareness of and resonance to the other's pain, with the intention to alleviate that pain to the best of one's ability, and from a self-state of metacognitive awareness, acceptance, and equanimity. It is a skill and a set of intentions to be cultivated, through experiential exercises and practices. Fortunately, science and clinical practices are forming a meeting ground, out of which a number of compassion training programs have emerged (Germer, 2009; Gilbert, 2009a; Singer & Bolz, 2013; Tirch et al., 2014). The Singer and Bolz volume is available as a free, downloadable e-book, and it contains detailed protocols of existing compassion training programs. In turn, one can contact the training centers for further information about workshops and other training opportunities. My own practice includes the following, at the beginning of each day in my clinic. I customarily sit in my consultation room in the cancer center, door closed, with one lamp on. I adopt a posture of mindful awareness, sitting as I teach others to do, in a comfortable and dignified manner, with a half-smile, hands gently upturned, palms open, breathing in, belly first:

1. Today, I am bringing my A-game to the people who are coming to me for help, and I trust that we will find a way together to ease their suffering.
2. I am willing to hold the pain and suffering of those who ask for my help today, making room for my own history of pain, knowing that some of it may show up here today.
3. I am grateful to my teachers, in life and in my practice, for the knowledge and skills they gave me.
4. Breathing in: compassion, lightheartedness, bravery. Breathing out: compassion, lightheartedness, bravery, to everyone in the clinic today: myself, the housekeeping staff, lab technicians, administrators, the front desk staff, the nurses and medical assistants, physicians assistants, doctors, the patients, and their loved ones.

I keep the list of statements on a card in my briefcase. Some days I recite them word for word; some days I just take a few moments to connect to the intentions behind the words. There are other days when perhaps only one of these points is especially salient. I don't just do this for my patients and their families; I do it for my own well-being also. And with that, I am off to see the day's patients.

A Focus on Strengths, Values, and Well-Being

Just as we draw on the strengths and values of our patients, to help them create meaning and well-being in the midst of challenges, we want to use the same tools for ourselves. The therapist is well served by taking a few minutes to review the adaptation of the Valued Living Questionnaire (Wilson et al., 2010), which was introduced in Chapter 6, on the treatment of depression.

Take the time now to study the values domains and to rate the importance of each to you. Think in terms of how these values support your efforts to be of service to cancer patients. And consider the values in light of what supports not only good care of others but also good, compassionate care of yourself. Now set the questionnaire aside for a moment. We will return to it later, when we design an action plan. Consider that our efforts to care for others are enhanced when we care for ourselves. Findings from the new neuroscience of compassion suggest that states of well-being and equanimity, with reasonable regulation of intense emotions, are conducive to compassionate care, and to creativity in-the-moment. These are ways of being (Bennett-Levy et al., 2015) that can potentially be built, in the same disciplined way that we might build muscle mass by lifting weights; psychotherapy skills by study, training, being observed and rated by expert practitioners; or musicianship by practice and guidance from teachers and mentors.

What if we can create strategies to build on therapist strengths and values, in order to purposefully build self-processes or ways of being that support not only our work but our own well-being? Isn't this, in essence, precisely what we are offering to our patients?

The path to creating more flexible, present-centered, engaged, and value-led self-states is not through ridding ourselves of our histories, our thoughts, or our painful emotional and behavioral repertoires. Our histories are not subtracted, and many forms of CBT, and the science underlying CBT, know this (Teasdale, 1999; Brewin, 2006; Hayes, Strosahl, & Wilson, 2012; Korrelboom et al., 2012; Korrelboom et al., 2013; Segal et al., 2013; Bennett-Levy et al., 2015). We can learn to make room, gently and persistently, for our historical repertoire of thoughts, images, body sensations, memories, emotions, and action patterns, without making them the enemy or fighting with them. They can just be there, in a space of acceptance and openness, held by a wise, observing self, who is freer to choose what to do right now. If so, consider the ways of being, including perspectives, postures, body sensations, and especially actions, that would support you in creating a newer way of being in the world. One model for self-practice and self-reflection is available in Bennett-Levy et al. (2015). I will draw on the model we have used in this book for our patients to help you design a strategy to experiment with in your own lives (exercise, spiritual practices, literature, music, creative work, gratitude practices).

Connecting to Context

We have seen that humans are tribal and highly dependent upon social context, for love, validation, and survival. Self-in-context is not isolated. Many of the strategies for working briefly with depressed and anxious cancer patients involved helping them access social support, develop perspective-taking ability about others in their lives, and engage more effectively with the people in their lives, from the medical teams to their loved ones. Limited social contexts portend poorer outcomes, emotionally, and in terms of psychophysiological markers of distress. The same is true of us. One potential role of the behavioral health consultant in cancer care teams is to facilitate the humanistic side of care, not only for the patients but also for one another on the team. Ideally, medical oncology teams function similarly to consultations teams in DBT, in the sense that caring for one another, assessing and helping to reduce burnout, and building team rapport and shared commitment can help improve patient care as well as staff well-being. In settings that do not foster larger team camaraderie, the behavioral health clinician will need to find at least one or two like-minded team members with whom to create a support team. In addition, opportunities for case consultation and clinical skill building need to be a part of the ongoing development of the behavioral health professional.

In taking another look at your values questionnaire, make a note of the people who can support you, and who you can support, in bringing your behavior more in line with what matters to you. If there are thorny relationship problems, job dissatisfaction, self-limiting and damaging therapeutic beliefs, physical well-being challenges, limited exercise or movement, overwork that impedes access to recreation and fun, an absence of spiritual growth, these areas of life may be affecting not only your well-being, but eventually, your work. They are areas to nurture, and one way to do so is through careful cultivation of our intentions, the purposeful development of self-processes, and by accessing and building social support for our intentions.

Creating an Action Plan: Dealing with a Specific Work Challenge

All of us face challenges in our work, and we can use the tools of our model to address those challenges. Let yourself focus on a challenge you face, either with a case, or with another aspect of the workplace. See if the vicious cycle model can help you map your own response to the challenge.

Allow yourself to think through what activating event seems implicated in this situation. Notice what thoughts and/or images emerge in response to this activating event. Notice the body sensations and emotions that arise as you enter this cycle of responding. What action urges and behaviors occur? With what consequences, to you and perhaps others in this situation? Notice if this has the quality of a game without end, in the sense that it recurs, and appears to take on a life of its own, as though you are caught on automatic pilot here. Now take a moment to become present to your sense of self, noticing the "me" that shows up in this cycle. Take a few minutes to fill in the cycle, in writing.

Here is an example from another therapist, Janelle, an experienced clinical psychologist, who has worked with cancer patients for the past 5 years, but has been with the new team just for 8 months.

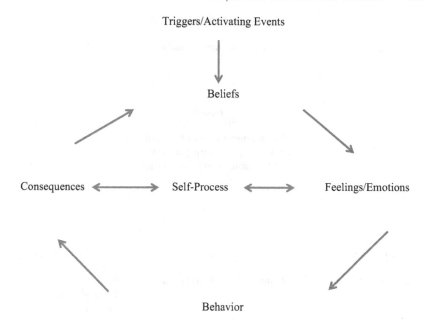

Triggers/Activating Events

Beliefs

Consequences ⟷ Self-Process ⟷ Feelings/Emotions

Behavior

FIGURE 9.1 Vicious or Virtuous Cycles

Adapted from: F. Wills (2015). *Skills in Cognitive Behaviour Therapy (2nd Edition)*, London: Sage.

From the vicious cycle that Janelle filled out, we can see that an apparent conflict with one of the medical oncologists has served as an activating event for the vicious cycle. Specifically, she noted that Dr. X is demanding and insensitive, not only of his patients but also his team, of which Janelle now serves as the behavioral health consultant. In morning rounds recently, Dr. X appeared distant and rather dismissive of Janelle's efforts with one patient who the team regarded to be particularly challenging. The patient has features of borderline personality disorder, and her chaotic lifestyle and explosive emotional outburst were highly off-putting to Dr. X. In rounds, Dr. X seemed to be upset with Janelle for not more rapidly ending the spate of demanding phone calls from the patient and teaching the patient to collaborate more effectively with the team. Janelle has ruminated about rounds and has become increasingly angry, scared and physically tense. Her sleep is affected, and she is starting to dread morning rounds. She has avoided talking directly with Dr. X and recently caught herself complaining about him to other team members, all of whom share her views of Dr. X. She is aware that this pattern is harming not only the team but also is creating a self-perpetuating state of being in which she feels diminished, weak, and ineffectual. She recognizes this pattern as old, in terms of her life history. Yet she is determined to do something to change this situation, for herself, and for the well-being of the team.

Janelle took a look at her beliefs about Dr. X and about herself. While there was some possibility that he might be upset with her, and quit referring, she believed,

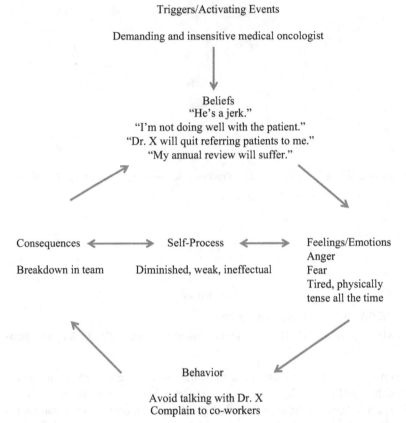

Triggers/Activating Events

Demanding and insensitive medical oncologist

Beliefs
"He's a jerk."
"I'm not doing well with the patient."
"Dr. X will quit referring patients to me."
"My annual review will suffer."

Consequences ⟷ Self-Process ⟷ Feelings/Emotions
                                          Anger
Breakdown in team   Diminished, weak, ineffectual   Fear
                                          Tired, physically
                                          tense all the time

Behavior

Avoid talking with Dr. X
Complain to co-workers

FIGURE 9.2 Vicious Cycle: Janelle

Adapted from: F. Wills (2015). *Skills in Cognitive Behaviour Therapy (2nd Edition)*. London: Sage.

after reflection, that her position was secure. She also recognized that other patients such as the one in question tended to provoke a strong response in Dr. X. Janelle's own sense of vulnerability was perhaps overblown, and in some ways related to her early life history, including possible core beliefs arising in the context of her family of origin. She sought consultation with a colleague, a senior psychologist whom she trusted, and came up with the following plan, intended to break up the budding vicious cycle of avoidance, fear, anger, worry, and physical tension, and to do her best to experience self as an effective presence. She set up a time for a brief private conversation with Dr. X. Though she was scared when she spoke to him, she learned that he, too, felt at times inadequate to help this particular patient, angry with the patient, then guilty for being angry. He acknowledged that he was hoping that Janelle would change the patient rapidly, as this was somehow his expectation for what psychologists and other behavioral health consultants were supposed to do. Janelle shared with Dr. X that she, too, felt put upon, and feared that she would not be seen to be doing her job. However, she explained the nature of borderline personality to him and helped him recognize that such patients often have anguished lives, which compound their coping challenges when they are faced with cancer. She set realistic expectations, including how the team could set up boundaries on phone calls and basic strategies for managing emotion dysregulation by the patient when she came in for follow-up. No quick cures were in sight. A more modest behavioral health agenda was crafted. And Janelle and Dr. X left the meeting agreeing that they had deepened their understanding of one another and their roles on the team. Taking things a bit further, Janelle spoke with the two other team members, to whom she had complained about Dr. X. She explained that she had developed a different understanding of Dr. X's motives and character and that she was committed to working effectively with all team members, rather than supporting a pattern of office gossip and ineffective problem solving. She emerged from the experience with a strengthened sense of self as effective, powerful, and able to manage her own inner turmoil more effectively in relation to her work team. The makings of a virtuous cycle were in place.

Now let's return to the Vicious Cycle you filled out for the work-related challenge you face. See if any of the beliefs about self and work that you filled out earlier in this chapter show up in the vicious cycle. Now, let's turn to creating a Virtuous Cycle out of the work-related problem you identified earlier.

Begin by letting yourself settle into your chair, sitting in a comfortable position, body in a dignified position, back straight enough for your breath to fill the belly,

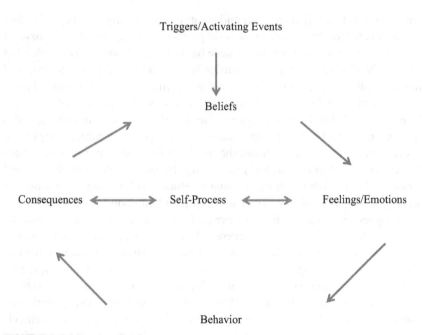

FIGURE 9.3 Virtuous Cycle

Adapted from: F. Wills (2015). *Skills in Cognitive Behaviour Therapy (2nd Edition)*. London: Sage.

then gently lift the diaphragm upward as air flows into the top of the lungs. Allowing yourself to feel the gravity pulling your body against the chair, and the floor, let yourself imagine being the self you wish to be in this situation. Bring some compassion to yourself, and notice the effects on your mind, emotions, and body of the situation you are in. From that place of seeing how this might play out, take a few moments to return to the book, and to the Virtuous Cycle.

Are there any other ways of viewing the situation you are in? Are there possibly other explanations that may not only fit the facts but also serve you better, not only in managing this situation but also in being who you wish to be in this and related situations? Can you carry the emotions along with you, gently and with caring for the pain? Notice the body sensations and consider what messages the emotions and body sensations may be conveying to you. Think through a fresh strategy you might embark on to bring either a different outcome or to cope with the emotions and thoughts that arise if no different outcome is feasible right now. Write down your answers on the form. Think about committing to implementing a change or acceptance strategy, wholeheartedly, and with an experimental eye: see what difference it makes, not only in terms of the consequences of being caught in this cycle but also for the sense of self you wish to increasingly embody.

Creating a Plan to Build States of Well-Being

Janelle took to heart what her body and emotions were telling her. She had let fear and avoidance trump her otherwise solid problem-solving skills. On the basis of the results of her values inventory, Janelle began to reflect on the need to develop a more effective long-term plan to manage her life, in relation to the challenges of working with cancer patients. From time spent with the values inventory, Janelle realized that several domains in her life were important but had not been sufficiently attended to for many months: her health, her key relationships, and a sense of fun had all gone missing in action over the past 8 months. Perhaps in an effort to prove herself to the team, she had been forgoing opportunities to have fun, even on her days off. She had given up regular exercise, although she was well aware of the research literature showing its efficacy in lowering depression and anxiety and in increasing states of well-being and emotion regulation. She was spending less time with friends, and her husband had been complaining that she was becoming less responsive and interested, sexually, and generally as a companion. Janelle committed to writing a detailed plan to address these areas of her life. She began by imagining in vivid detail and walking through steps she could take to modestly re-engage with exercise and with recreational activities. She imagined her sense of self in relation to her husband as she took steps to re-engage with him, convinced that work, and not other marital problems, were the primary difficulties. Finally, she started a morning well-being check-in with her team members, in which she and others had the chance to share a poem, a meditation, a prayer, a worry about a patient, a clinical challenge. This deepening of her spiritual life and team involvement was satisfying. One morning, Dr. X brought a poem on healing that had moved him recently, and he read it aloud to the team.

Among the commitments she made to herself, were the following:

Action Plan for Managing the Mind

Janelle committed to checking facts when she noticed that she jumped to painful conclusions. She also committed to trusting herself: that if her painful conclusions were accurate, she would find a productive way to deal with life as it is. She also decided to sign up for a Mindfulness-Based Stress Reduction program, to cultivate and practice the skill of non-judgmentally observing what arises in the mind, emotions, and body. She also began reading and watching some YouTube videos about compassion focused approaches to self-care, as she was increasingly aware that she had a harsh inner critic that spilled over into self-damaging behavioral strategies at times. Noticing how her mind leaned toward the critical, in herself and others, Janelle committed to briefly noting two or three things, once a week, for which she could experience gratitude. She bought a small notebook, which she kept on her night stand, and dated the entries she made. She decided to confine her gratitude practice, for now, to work-related matters. She was surprised, after a month, to discover the number of other people and experiences at work, for which she was grateful.

Action Plan for Physical and Emotional Well-Being

Janelle's values worksheet showed her the importance of protecting her own health. She committed to a small but realistic step toward increasing exercise. She brought some walking shoes to work and found a colleague with whom she could begin taking 20-minute walks, twice a week. She had thought about resuming yoga classes but decided that committing to the walks was the most realistic step for now. She committed to brief, weekly massages at a massage station in the hospital. She also committed to time each work night, to light a candle and sit with her husband, listening to soothing and contemplative music together. Finally, rather than watch cable news each evening, which both she and her husband agreed was more inflammatory than informative, Janelle got an anthology of poetry by one of her favorite writers, and read one poem after listening to music.

Action Plan for Connecting to Social Contexts

Janelle's values worksheet made her aware that she had begun to isolate from sources of love and support. She committed to increasing pleasurable time with her husband, including sharing with him in strategies for body and emotions. She committed to calling a cherished friend and resuming contact after many months. In her workplace, Janelle renewed a commitment to teaching and supervising. One of Janelle's strengths as a professional was her commitment to lifelong

learning. She was a valued mentor to graduate students, where she offered prac-
tica in CBT for cancer patients and families. She also shared her Well-Being Plan
with a colleague at work, making a verbal commitment and seeking her colleague's
support in carrying out her action plan. A month later, her colleague presented
his own Well-Being Plan to Janelle and asked for her support as well. As we saw
earlier, Janelle also took the step of implementing a morning consultation, which
included elements of professional and personal well-being for the entire oncology
team, on a voluntary basis. The meeting soon became a highly regarded mainstay
in the daily functioning of the team.

Let's close out this chapter, and this book, by having you prepare your own
Well-Being Plan. Take a moment to settle into a chair, reflecting on what life values and directions are calling you forward in your professional and personal life.
If you wish to, you might take a moment to close your eyes, contacting the wise
and compassionate space within that you extend to your patients. See if that self
is contained within the boundaries of your own skin, or if it extends beyond your
skin, your bones. Project forward in time, perhaps 3 years, and allow that wise
and compassionate self to take stock of you, now, in the chair. Perhaps a message
can emerge from that wise future self, suggesting how a Well-Being Plan might
look. Imagine being that plan. Let yourself form vivid images of yourself living
a well-being plan and experiencing the state of being implicit in the living. Now,
coming back to this moment, see if you can find the intention to make it so.

Take the time to write out a plan, limiting it to what you can commit to with at
least a 90% certainty of accomplishing over the coming month. If at the end of the
month, you wish to renew your commitment, do so. List someone you can share
these intentions with:

Name of my partner in well-being: _____

_____

Action plan for managing the mind: _____

_____

_____

_____

_____

Action plan for physical and emotional well-being: _____

_____

_____

_____

Action plan for connecting to social contexts: _____

_____

_____

_____

Appendix

**Edmonton Symptom
Assessment System
(ESAS-FS)**
Outpatient

Patien
ACCT#
DOB

Date:_____ Time:_____

In the last 24 hours on average I have felt:

Please circle the number that best describes your symptoms:

No Pain	0 1 2 3 4 5 6 7 8 9 10	Worst Pain
No Fatigue	0 1 2 3 4 5 6 7 8 9 10	Worst Fatigue
No Nausea	0 1 2 3 4 5 6 7 8 9 10	Worst Nausea
No Depression	0 1 2 3 4 5 6 7 8 9 10	Worst Depression
No Anxiety	0 1 2 3 4 5 6 7 8 9 10	Worst Anxiety
No Drowsiness	0 1 2 3 4 5 6 7 8 9 10	Worst Drowsiness
No Shortness of Breath	0 1 2 3 4 5 6 7 8 9 10	Worst Shortness of Breath
Best Appetite	0 1 2 3 4 5 6 7 8 9 10	Worst Appetite
Best Feeling of Well Being	0 1 2 3 4 5 6 7 8 9 10	Worst Feeling of Well Being
Best Sleep	0 1 2 3 4 5 6 7 8 9 10	Worst Sleep
No Financial Distress *(Distress/suffering experienced secondary to financial issues)*	0 1 2 3 4 5 6 7 8 9 10	Worst Financial Distress
No Spiritual Pain *(Pain deep in your soul/being that is not physical)*	0 1 2 3 4 5 6 7 8 9 10	Worst Spiritual Pain

Completed by: ☐ Patient   ☐ Family

Assessed by (Signature/Credentials/ID#/ Date/ Time)_____
Print / Stamp Name: _____

References

Aderka, I., Nickerson, A., Boe, K., & Hofmann, S. (2012). Sudden gains during psychological treatments of anxiety and depression: a meta-analysis. *Journal of Consulting and Clinical Psychology*, 80: 93–101.

American Cancer Society. (2012). *Cancer treatment and survivorship facts and figures 2012–2013*. Atlanta, GA: American Cancer Society.

American Cancer Society. (2014). *Cancer facts and figures, 7*. Atlanta, GA: American Cancer Society.

American Psychiatric Association. (2013). *Diagnostic and statistical manual of mental disorders (5th Edition)*. Washington, DC: Author.

Anda, R., Butchart, A., Felitti, V., & Brown, D. (2010). Building a framework for global surveillance of the public health implications of adverse childhood experiences. *American Journal of Preventive Medicine*, 39 (1): 93–98.

Antoni, M. (2003). *Stress management intervention for women with breast cancer*. Washington, DC: American Psychological Association Press.

Antoni, M., Lehman, J.M., Kilbourn, K.M., Boyers, A.E., Culver, J.L., Alferi, S.M., . . . Carver, C.S. (2001). Cognitive-behavioral stress management intervention decreases the prevalence of depression and enhances benefit finding among women under treatment for early-stage breast cancer. *Health Psychology*, January, 20 (1): 20–32.

Arch, J. & Mitchell, J. (2016). An Acceptance and Commitment Therapy group intervention for cancer survivors experiencing anxiety at re-entry. *Psycho-Oncology*, 25 (5): 610–615.

Baer, R. (2014). *Mindfulness-based treatment approaches: clinician's guide to evidence based and applications (2nd Edition)*. London: Elsevier.

Baer, R. & Walsh, E. (2016). Treating acute depression with mindfulness-based cognitive therapy. In *Treating depression: MCT, CBT and Third Wave Therapies*, 344–368 (A. Wells & P. Fisher, Eds.). West Sussex, UK: John Wiley & Sons.

Baker, P., Beesley, H., Dinwoodie, R., Fletcher, I., Ablett, J., Holcombe, C., & Salmon, P. (2013). 'You're putting thoughts into my head': a qualitative study of readiness of patients with breast, lung or prostate cancer to address emotional needs through the first 18 months after diagnosis. *Psycho-Oncology*, 22: 1402–1410.

Barlow, D., Allen, L., & Choate, M. (2004). Towards a unified treatment for emotional disorders. *Behavior Therapy*, 35: 205–230.

Bartley, T. (2012). *Mindfulness-based cognitive therapy for cancer*. London: Wiley-Blackwell.

Bateman, A. & Fonagy, P. (Eds.). (2012). *Handbook of mentalizing in mental health practice*. Washington, DC: American Psychiatric Publishing.

Beck, A. (1996). Beyond belief: a theory of modes, personality, and psychopathology. In *Frontiers of cognitive therapy*, 1–25 (P. Salkovskis, Ed.). New York: Guilford Press.

Beck, A., Davis, D., & Freeman, A. (2006). *Cognitive therapy of personality disorders (3rd Edition)*. New York: Guilford Press.

Beck, A. & Dozois, D. (2011). Cognitive therapy: current status and future directions. *Annual Review of Medicine*, 62: 397–409.

Beck, A. & Emery, G. (1985). *Anxiety disorders and phobias: a cognitive perspective*. New York: Basic Books.

Beck, A. & Haigh, E. (2014). Advances in cognitive theory and therapy: the generic cognitive model. *Annual Review of Clinical Psychology*, 10: 1–24.

Beck, A. & Rush, J. (1979). *Cognitive therapy of depression*. New York: Guilford Press.

Beck, J. (1995). *Cognitive therapy: basics and beyond*. New York: Guilford Press.

Beck, J. (2011a). *Cognitive therapy: basics and beyond (2nd Edition)*. New York: Guilford Press.

Beck, J. (2011b). *Cognitive therapy for challenging problems: what to do when the basics don't work*. New York: Guilford Press.

Bennett-Levy, J., Butler, G., Fennell, M., Hackmann, A., Mueller, M., & Westbrook, D. (2004). *Oxford guide to behavioural experiments in cognitive therapy*. Oxford: Oxford University Press.

Bennett-Levy, J., Thwaites, R., Haarhoff, B., & Perry, H. (2015). *Experiencing CBT from the inside out: a self-practice/self-reflection workbook for therapists*. New York: Guilford Press.

Borkovec, T.D. (2006). Applied relaxation and cognitive therapy for pathological worry and generalized anxiety disorder. In *Worry and its psychological disorders: theory, assessment and treatment*, 273–288 (G.C.L. Davey and A. Wells, Eds.). Chichester, UK: John Wiley & Sons.

Boszormenyi-Nagy, I. & Krasner, B. (1986). *Between give and take: a clinical guide to contextual therapy.* New York: Brunner/Mazel.

Breitbart, W. & Poppito, S. (2014). *Individual meaning-centered psychotherapy for patients with advanced cancer: a treatment manual.* Oxford: Oxford University Press.

Breitbart, W., Rosenfeld, B., Gibson, C., Pessin, H., Poppito, S., Nelson, C., . . . Olden, M. (2010). Meaning-centered group psychotherapy for patients with advanced cancer: a pilot randomized controlled trial. *Psycho-Oncology,* 19 (1): 21–28.

Brewin, C. (2006). Understanding cognitive behavior therapy: a retrieval competition account. *Behaviour Research and Therapy,* 44: 765–784.

Brintzenhofe-Szoc, K., Levin, T., Li, Y., Kissane, D., & Zabora, J. (2009). Mixed anxiety/depression symptoms in a large cancer cohort: prevalence by cancer type. *Psychosomatics,* 50 (4): 383–391.

Brown, D.W., Anda, R.F., Felitti, V.J., Edwards, V.J., Malarcher, A.M., Croft, J.B., & Giles, W.H. (2010). Adverse childhood experiences are associated with the risk of lung cancer: a prospective cohort study. *Public Health,* 10 (20). DOI: 10.1186/1471-2458-10-20.

Bruera, E. & MacDonald, S. (1993). Audit methods: the Edmonton symptom assessment system. In *Clinical audit in palliative care,* 61–77 (I. Higginson, Ed.). Oxford: Radcliffe Medical Press.

Budman, S. & Gurman, A. (2002). *Theory and practice of brief therapy.* New York: Guilford Press.

Butler, G., Fennell, M., & Hackmann, A. (2008). *Cognitive-behavioral therapy for anxiety disorders: mastering clinical challenges.* New York: Guilford Press.

Camus, A. (1955). *The myth of Sisyphus and other essays.* New York: Albert A. Knopf.

Capra, F. & Luisi, P. (2014). *The systems view of life: a unifying vision.* Cambridge: Cambridge University Press.

Carlson, L. & Speca, M. (2010). *Mindfulness-based cancer recovery.* Oakland, CA: New Harbinger Press.

Carver, C. & Antoni, M. (2004). Finding benefit in breast cancer during the year after diagnosis predicts better adjustment 5 to 8 years after diagnosis. *Health Psychology,* 23 (6): 595–598.

Chang, V., Hwang, S., & Feuerman, M. (2000). Validation of the Edmonton symptom assessment scale. *Cancer,* 88: 2164–2171.

Chödrön, P. (2001). *The places that scare you: a guide to fearlessness in difficult times.* Boulder, CO: Shambhala.

Clark, D.A. & Beck, A.T. (2010). *Cognitive therapy of anxiety disorders: science and practice.* New York: Guilford Press.

Clark, D.A. & Beck, A.T. (2012). *The anxiety and worry workbook: the cognitive behavioral solution.* New York: Guilford Press.

Clark, D.M. (1986). A cognitive approach to panic. *Behaviour Research and Therapy,* 24: 461–470.

Cohen, R., Bavashi, C., & Rozanski, A. (2016). Purpose in life and its relationship to all-cause mortality and cardiovascular events: a meta-analysis. *Psychosomatic Medicine*, 78 (2): 122–133.

Cook, S., Salmon, P., Holcombe, C., Cornford, P., Dunn, G., & Fisher, P. (2015). The association of metacognitive beliefs with emotional distress after diagnosis of cancer. *Health Psychology*, 34 (3): 207–215.

Cormier, H. (2001). *The truth is what works: William James, pragmatism, and the seed of death*. Lanham, MD: Rowman & Littlefield.

Corso, P., Edwards, V., Fange, X., & Mercy, J. (2008). Health-related quality of life among adults who experienced maltreatment during childhood. *American Journal of Public Health*, 98 (6): 1094–1100.

Crane, R. (2009). *Mindfulness-based cognitive therapy: distinctive features*. New York: Routledge/Taylor & Francis.

Dahl, J., Plumb, J., Stewart, I., & Lundgren, T. (2009). *The art and science of valuing in psychotherapy: helping clients discover, explore, and commit to valued action using acceptance and commitment therapy*. Oakland, CA: New Harbinger.

Davidson, R. & Begley, S. (2012). *The emotional life of your brain*. New York: Penguin Books.

Deacon, B., Sy, J., Lickel, J., & Nelson, E. (2010). Does the judicious use of safety behaviors improve the efficacy and acceptability for exposure therapy for claustrophobic fear? *Journal of Behavior Therapy and Experimental Psychiatry*, 41: 71–80.

deMoor, J., Mariotto, A., Parry, C., Alfano, C., Padgett, K., Kent, E., & Rowland, J. (2013). Cancer survivors in the United States: prevalence across the survivorship trajectory and implications for care. *Cancer Epidemiology, Biomarkers & Prevention*, 22: 561–570.

deShazar, S. (1988). *Clues: investigating solutions in brief therapy*. New York: W.W. Norton.

Didion, J. (2006). *We tell ourselves stories in order to live: collected nonfiction*. New York: Alfred A. Knopf.

Dimidjian, S., Hollon, S.D., Dobson, K.S., Schamling, K.B., Kohlenberg, R.J., Addis, M.E., . . . Jacobson, N.S.(2006). Randomized trial of behavioral activation, cognitive therapy, and antidepressant medication in the acute treatment of adults with major depression. *Journal of Consulting and Clinical Psychology*, 74 (4): 658–670.

Eells, T. (2015). *Psychotherapy case formulation*. Washington, DC: American Psychological Association.

Ehlers, A. & Clark, D. (2000). A cognitive model of posttraumatic stress disorder. *Behaviour Research and Therapy*, 38: 319–345.

Ehlers, A., Clark, D., Hackman, A., Grey, N., Liness, S., Wild, J., . . . Waddington, L. (2010). Intensive cognitive therapy for PTSD: a feasibility study. *Behavioural and Cognitive Psychotherapy*, 38: 383–398.

Eifert, G. & Forsyth, J. (2005). *Acceptance and commitment therapy for anxiety disorders: a practitioner's treatment guide*. Oakland, CA: New Harbinger Press.

Ekkers, W., Korrelboom, K., Huijbrechts, I., Smits, N., Cuijpers, P., & van der Gaag, M. (2011). Competitive memory training for treating depression and rumination in depressed older adults: a randomized controlled trial. *Behaviour Research and Therapy*, 49: 588–596.

Epston, D. & White, M. (1990). *Narrative means to therapeutic ends*. New York: W.W. Norton.

Feros, D., Lane, L., Ciarrochi, J., & Blackledge, J. (2013). Acceptance and Commitment Therapy (ACT) for improving the lives of cancer patients: a preliminary study. *Psycho-Oncology*, 22, 2, 459-464.

Figley, C. (Ed). (1995). *Compassion fatigue: coping with secondary trauma*. New York: Routledge/Taylor & Francis Group.

Fine, R. (1962, 2014). *Freud: a critical re-evaluation of his theories*. New York: Routledge.

Flechtner, H. & Bottomley, A. (2003). Fatigue and quality of life: lessons from the real world. *Oncologist*, 8 (Suppl 1): 5–9.

Forsey, M., Salmon, P., Eden, T., & Young, B. (2013). Comparing doctors' and nurses' accounts of how they provide emotional care for parents of children with acute lymphoblastic leukaemia. *Psycho-Oncology*, 22: 260–267.

Forsyth, J. & Eifert, G. (2008). *The mindfulness and acceptance workbook for anxiety: a guide to breaking free from anxiety, phobias, and worry*. Oakland, CA: New Harbinger.

Frankl, V. (1986). *The doctor and the soul: from psychotherapy to logotherapy*. New York: Vintage Books.

Frankl, V. (1992). *Man's search for meaning*. Boston: Beacon Press.

Freud, S. (1958). Papers on technique, 1910–1915. In *The standard edition of the complete psychological works of Sigmund Freud*, Vol. 22, London: Hogarth Press.

Friedman, M. (1991). *Encounter on the narrow ridge: a life of Martin Buber*. New York: Paragon House.

Garssen, B. (2004). Psychological factors and cancer development: evidence after 30 years of research. *Clinical Psychology Review*, 24: 315–338.

Gawande, A. (2015). *Being mortal*. New York: Henry Holt & Company.

Gehart, D. (2014). *Mastering competencies in family therapy (2nd Edition)*. Belmont, CA: Brooks/Cole.

Germer, C. (2009). *The mindful path to self-compassion: freeing yourself from destructive thoughts and emotions*. New York: Guilford Press.

Gilbert, P. (Ed). (2004). *Evolutionary therapy and cognitive therapy*. New York: Springer.

Gilbert, P. (2009a). *The compassionate mind*. London: Constable & Robinson.

Gilbert, P. (2009b). *Overcoming depression*. New York: Basic Books.

Gilbert, P. (2010). *Compassion focused therapy*. New York: Routledge/Taylor & Francis Group.

Gilbert, P. (2014). The origins and nature of compassion focused therapy. *British Journal of Clinical Psychology*, 53: 6–41.

Gilbert, P. & Choden, K. (2014). *Mindful compassion: using the power of mindfulness and compassion to transform our lives.* London: Constable & Robinson.

Gottman, J. & Levenson, R. (1992). Marital processes predictive of later dissolution: behavior, physiology, and health. *Journal of Personality and Social Psychology, 63* (2): 221–233.

Grabovac, A., Lau, M., & Willett, B. (2011). Mechanisms of mindfulness: a Buddhist psychological model. *Mindfulness, 2*: 154–166.

Greenberg, L. (2011). *Emotion-focused therapy.* Washington, DC: American Psychological Association.

Greenberger, D. & Padesky, C. (2015). *Mind over mood: change how you feel by changing the way you think (2nd Edition).* New York: Guilford Press.

Gustafson, J. (1986). *The complex secret of brief psychotherapy.* New York: W.W. Norton.

Gustafson, J. (1992). *Self-delight in a harsh world: the main stories of individual, marital, and family psychotherapy.* New York: W.W. Norton.

Gustafson, J. (2005). *Very brief psychotherapy.* New York: Routledge/Taylor & Frances.

Hackmann, A., Bennett-Levy, J., & Holmes, E. (2011). *Oxford guide to imagery in cognitive therapy.* Oxford: Oxford University Press.

Haidt, J. (2006). *The happiness hypothesis: finding modern truth in ancient wisdom.* New York: Basic Books.

Harding, R., Beesley, H., Holcombe, C., Fisher, J., & Salmon, P. (2015). Are patient-nurse relationships in breast cancer linked to adult attachment style? *Journal of Advanced Nursing, 71* (10): 2305–2314.

Hargrave, T. & Pfitzer, F. (2003). *The new contextual therapy: guiding the power of give and take.* New York: Brunner-Routledge Press.

Harvey, A., Watkins, E., Mansell, W., & Shafran, R. (2004). *Cognitive behavioural processes across psychological disorders.* Oxford: Oxford University Press.

Hawkes, A.L., Chambers, S.K., Pakenham, K.I., Patrao, T.A., Baade, P.D., Lynch, B.M., . . . Courneyea, K.S.(2013). Effects of a telephone-delivered multiple health behavior change intervention (CanChange) on health and behavioral outcomes in survivors of colorectal cancer: a randomized controlled trial. *Journal of Clinical Oncology, 31* (18): 2313–2321.

Hawkes, A., Pakenham, K., & Chambers, S. (2014). Effects of a multiple health behavior change intervention for colorectal cancer survivors on psychosocial outcomes and quality of life: a randomized controlled trial. *Annals of Behavioral Medicine, 48*: 359–370.

Hayes, S. (1984). Making sense of spirituality. *Behaviorism, 12*: 99–110.

Hayes, S. (2004). Acceptance and commitment therapy, relational frame theory, and the Third Wave of behavior therapy. *Behavior Therapy, 35*: 639–665.

Hayes, S. (2016). Perspective-taking as healing. In *The self-acceptance project: how to be kind and compassionate toward yourself in any situation*, 29–38 (T. Simon, Ed.). Boulder, CO: Sounds True.

Hayes, S., Barnes-Holmes, D., & Roche, B. (2001). *Relational frame theory: a post-Skinnerian account of human language and cognition*. New York: Plenum Press.

Hayes, S., Brownstein, A., Zettle, R., Rosenfarb, I., & Korn, Z. (1986). Rule-governed behavior and sensitivity to changing consequences of responding. *Journal of the Experimental Analysis of Behavior*, 45: 237–256.

Hayes, S., Follette, V., & Linehan, M. (Eds). (2004). *Mindfulness and acceptance: expanding the cognitive-behavioral tradition*. New York: Guilford Press.

Hayes, S., Hayes, L., Reese, H., & Sarbin, T. (Eds.). (1993). *Varieties of scientific contextualism*. Reno, NV: Context Press.

Hayes, S. & Sanford, B. (2014). Cooperation came first: evolution and human cognition. *Journal of the Experimental Analysis of Behavior*, 101: 112–129.

Hayes, S., Strosahl, K., & Wilson, K. (2012). *Acceptance and commitment therapy: the process and practice of mindful change (2nd Edition)*. New York: Guilford Press.

Hayes, S., Villatte, M., Levin, M., & Hildebrandt, M. (2011). Open, aware, and active: contextual approaches as an emerging trend in behavioral and cognitive therapies. *Annual Review of Clinical Psychology*, 7: 141–168.

Herbert, J. & Foreman, E. (2011). *Acceptance and mindfulness in cognitive-behavior therapy: understanding and applying the new therapies*. Hoboken: John Wiley & Sons.

Herbert, J., Forman, E., & Hitchcock, P. (2016). Contextual approaches to psychotherapy: defining, distinguishing and common features. In *The Wiley handbook of contextual behavioral science*, 287–302 (R.D. Zettle, S.C. Hayes, D. Barnes-Holmes & A. Biglan, Eds.). Malden, MA: Wiley Blackwell.

Heuman, L. (2014). The embodied mind: an interview with philosopher Evan Thompson. *Tricycle*, Fall.

Hill, J., Holcombe, C., Clark, L., Boothby, M., Hincks, A., Fisher, J., . . . Salmon, P. (2011). Predictors of onset of depression and anxiety in the year after diagnosis of breast cancer. *Psychological Medicine*, 41: 1429–1436.

Hofmann, S.G. (2011). Loving-kindness and compassion meditation: potential for psychological interventions. *Clinical Psychology Review*, 31 (7): 1126–1132.

Hofmann, S.G. (2012). *An introduction to modern CBT*. West Sussex: Wiley-Blackwell.

Hofmann, S.G., Petrocchi, N., Steinberg, J., Lin, M., Arimitsu, K., Kind, S., . . . Stangier, U. (2015). Loving-kindness meditation to target affect in mood disorders: a proof-of-concept study. *Evidence-Based Complementary and Alternative Medicine*, 2015: Article ID 269126, 11 pages. DOI: http://dx.doi.org/10.1155/2015/269126.

Holland, J. (2002). History of psycho-oncology: overcoming attitudinal and conceptual barriers. *Psychosomatic Medicine*, 64: 206–221.

Hopko, D., Armento, M., Robertson, S., Ryba, M., Carvalho, J., Colman, L., . . . Lejuez, C.(2011). Brief behavioral activation and problem-solving therapy for depressed breast cancer patients: a randomized controlled trial. *Journal of Consulting and Clinical Psychology*, December, 79 (6): 834–849.

Hopko, D., Bell, J., Armento, M., Robertson, S., Mullane, C., Wolf, N., & Lejuez, C. (2008). Cognitive-behavior therapy for depressed cancer patients in a medical setting. *Behavior Therapy*, June, 39 (2): 126–136.

Hopko, D., Lejuez, C., Ruggiero, K., & Eifert, G. (2003). Contemporary behavioral activation treatments for depression: procedures, principles, and progress. *Clinical Psychology Review*, 23: 699–717.

Hoyt, M. & Talmon, M. (2014). *Capturing the moment: single session therapy and walk-in services.* Bethel, CT: Crown House.

Jacobson, N.S., Dobson, K.S., Truax, P.A., Addis, M.E., Koerner, K., Gollan, J.K., … Prince, S.E. (1996). A component analysis of cognitive-behavioral treatment of depression. *Journal of Consulting and Clinical Psychology*, 64 (2): 295–304.

Jacobsen, P. & Andrykowski, M. (2015). Tertiary prevention in cancer care: understanding and addressing the psychological dimensions of cancer during the active treatment period. *American Psychologist*, 70 (2): 134–145.

Jacobsen, P., Donovan, K.A., Trask, P.C., Fleishman, S.B., Zabora, J., Baker, F., & Holland, J.C. (2005). Screening for psychologic distress in ambulatory cancer patients. *Cancer*, April 1, 103 (7): 1494–1502.

James, W. (1890). The principles of psychology: the briefer course. In *William James: writings, 1878–1899* (G.E. Myers, Ed.). New York: Library of America.

Kabat-Zinn, J. (2013). *Full catastrophe living.* New York: Random House.

Kahneman, D. (2011). *Thinking fast and slow.* New York: Farrar, Straus and Giroux.

Kalanithi, P. (2016). *When breath becomes air.* New York: Random House.

Kazantzis, N., Fairburn, C., Padesky, C., Reinecke, M., & Teesson, M. (2014). Unresolved issues regarding the research and practice of cognitive behavior therapy: the case of guided discovery using Socratic questioning. *Behaviour Change*, 31 (1): 1–17.

Keefe, J. & DeRubeis, R. (2016). A critique of theoretical models of depression: commonalities and distinctive features. In *Treating depression: MCT, CBT and Third Wave therapies*, 242–262 (A. Wells & P. Fisher, Eds.). West Sussex, UK: John Wiley & Sons.

Kessler, R., Berglund, P., Demler, O., Jin, R., Merkiangas, K., & Walters, E. (2005). Lifetime Prevalence and Age-of-Onset Distributions of DSM-IV Disorders in the National Comorbidity Survey Replication, Archives of General Psychiatry, 62, 593–602.

Koerner, K. (2012). *Doing dialectical behavior therapy: a practical guide.* New York: Guilford Press.

Korrelboom, K., Maarsing, M., & Huijbrechts, I. (2012). Competitive memory training (COMET) for treating low self-esteem in patients with depressive disorders: a randomized clinical trial. *Depression and Anxiety*, February, 29 (2): 102–110.

Korrelboom, K., Peeters, S., Blom, S., & Huijbrechts, I. (2013). Competitive memory training (COMET) for panic and applied relaxation (AR) are equally effective in the treatment of panic in panic-disordered patients. *Journal of Contemporary Psychotherapy*, 44 (3). DOI 10.1007/s10879–013–9259–3

Kuyken, W., Padesky, C., & Dudley, R. (2009). *Collaborative case conceptualization: working effectively with clients in cognitive-behavioural therapy.* New York: Guilford Press.

Kuyken, W., Watkins, E., Holden, E., White, K., Taylor, R., Byford, S., . . . Dalgleish, T. (2010). How does mindfulness-based cognitive therapy work? *Behaviour Research and Therapy,* 48: 1105–1112.

Langer, E. (2014). *Mindfulness.* Philadelphia: DaCapo Press.

Lau, M. & McMain, S. (2005). Integrating mindfulness meditation with cognitive and behavioural therapies: the challenge of combining acceptance-and-change-based strategies. *Canadian Journal of Psychiatry,* November (50): 863–869.

Lau, M., Segal, Z., & Williams, M. (2004). Teasdale's differential activation hypothesis: implications for mechanisms of depressive relapse and suicidal behavior. *Behaviour Research and Therapy,* 42: 1001–1017.

Lazarus, R. & Folkmann, S. (1984). *Stress, appraisal, and coping.* New York: Springer.

Leahy, R. (2001). *Overcoming resistance in cognitive therapy.* New York: Guilford Press.

Leahy, R. (2006). *The worry cure: seven steps to stop worry from stopping you.* New York: Harmony Books.

Leahy, R. (2016). A critique of therapeutic approaches to depression: commonalities and distinctive features. In *Treating depression: MCT, CBT and Third Wave therapies,* 393–413(A. Wells & P. Fisher, Eds.). West Sussex, UK: John Wiley & Sons.

Leahy, R., Holland, S., & McGinn, L. (2011). *Treatment plans and interventions for depression and anxiety disorders.* New York: Guilford Press.

Levenson, H. (2010). *Brief dynamic therapy.* Washington, DC: American Psychological Association Press.

Levin, T. & Applebaum, A. (2012). Acute cancer cognitive therapy. *Cognitive and Behavioral Practice,* 21: 404–415.

Levin, T. & Kissane, D. (2006). Psychooncology: the state of its development in 2006. *European Journal of Psychiatry,* 20 (3): 183–197.

Levin, T., Riskind, J., & Li, Y. (2010). Looming cognitive style and quality of life in a cancer cohort. *Palliative and Supportive Care,* 28; 8 (4): 449–454.

Levin, T., White, C., Bialer, P., Charlson, R., & Kissane, D. (2013). A review of cognitive therapy in acute medical settings: part II: strategies and complexities. *Palliative and Supportive Care,* 11 (3): 253–266.

Levin, T., White, C., & Kissane, D. (2013). A review of cognitive therapy in acute medical settings: part I: therapy model and assessment. *Palliative and Supportive Care,* 11 (2): 141–153.

Levy, H. & Radomsky, A. (2014). Safety behavior enhances the acceptability of exposure. *Cognitive & Behavioural Therapies,* 43 (1): 83–92.

Li, M., Fitzgerald, P., & Rodin, G. (2012). Evidence-based treatment of depression in patients with cancer. *Journal of Clinical Oncology,* 30 (11): 1187–1196.

Lindblad-Goldberg, M., Dore, M., & Stern, L. (1989). *Creating competence from chaos: a comprehensive guide to home-based services.* New York: W.W. Norton.

Linehan, M. (1993a). *Cognitive behavior therapy for borderline personality disorder.* New York: Guilford Press.

Linehan, M. (1993b). *Skills training manual for treating borderline personality disorder.* New York: Guilford Press.

Linehan, M. (1997). Validation and psychotherapy. In *Empathy reconsidered: new directions in psychotherapy,* 353–392 (A. Bohart & L. Greenberg, Eds.). Washington, DC: American Psychological Association Press.

Linehan, M. (2015). *DBT skills training manual (2nd Edition).* New York: Guilford Press.

Longmore, R. & Worrell, M. (2007). Do we need to challenge thoughts in cognitive behavior therapy? *Clinical Psychology Review,* March, 27 (2): 173–187.

Lutgendorf, S. & Anderson, B. (2015). Biobehavioral approaches to cancer progression and survival: mechanisms and interventions. *American Psychologist,* February-March, 70 (2): 186–197.

Lyubomirsky, S. (2007). *The how of happiness: a new approach to getting the life you want.* New York: Penguin Books.

Lyubomirsky, S. (2013). *The myths of happiness.* New York: Penguin Books.

Mansell, W., Carey, T., & Tai, S. (2013). *A transdiagnostic approach to CBT using method of levels therapy.* East Sussex, UK: Routledge/Taylor Francis Group.

MAPPG. Mindfulness All-Party Parliamentary Group Interim Report. (2015).

Martell, C., Addis, M., & Jacobson, N. (2001). *Depression in context: strategies for guided action.* New York: W.W. Norton.

Martell, C., Dimidjian, S., & Herman-Dunn, R. (2010). *Behavioral activation for depression: a clinician's guide.* New York and London: Guilford Press.

Massie, M. (2004). Prevalence of depression in patients with cancer. *Journal of the National Cancer Institute Monographs,* 32: 57–71.

May, G. (1982). *Will and spirit: a contemplative psychology.* San Francisco: Harper & Row.

McDaniel, S., Doherty, W., & Hepworth, J. (2013). *Medical family therapy and integrated care (2nd Edition).* Washington, DC: American Psychological Association.

McHugh, L. & Stewart, I. (Eds). (2012). *The self and perspective taking: contributions and applications from modern behavioral science.* Reno: Context Press.

McManus, F., Van Doorn, K., & Yiend, J. (2011). Examining the effects of thought records and behavioral experiments in instigating belief change. *Journal of Behavior Therapy and Experimental Psychiatry,* 43, 540–547.

Meyer, T.J., Miller, M.L., Metzger, R.L., & Borkovec, T.D. (1990). Development and validation of the Penn State Worry Questionnaire. *Behaviour Research and Therapy,* 28: 487–495.

Minuchin, S. (1974). *Families and family therapy.* Cambridge, MA: Harvard University Press.

Minuchin, S. & Fishman, H. (1981). *Family therapy techniques.* Cambridge, MA: Harvard University Press.

Minuchin, S., Rosman, B., & Baker, L. (1978). *Psychosomatic families: anorexia nervosa in context.* Cambridge, MA: Harvard University Press.

Misono, S., Weiss, N.S., Fann, J.R., Redman, M., Yueh, B. (2008). Incidence of suicide in persons with cancer. *Journal of Clinical Oncology*, 26 (29): 4731–4738.

Mitchell, A., Chan, M., Bhatti, H., Halton, M., Grassi, L., Johansen, C., & Meader, N. (2011). Prevalence of depression, anxiety, and adjustment disorder in oncological, haematological, and palliative-care settings: a meta-analysis of 94 interview-based studies. *Lancet Oncology*, 12: 160–174.

Mitchell, A., Ferguson, D., Gill, J., Paul, J., & Symonds, P. (2013). Depression and anxiety in long-term cancer survivors compared with spouses and healthy controls: a systematic review and meta-analysis. *Lancet Oncology*, 14: 721–732.

Moorey, S. & Greer, S. (2012). *Oxford guide to CBT for people with cancer*. Oxford: Oxford University Press.

Mukherjee, S. (2010). *The emperor of all maladies: a biography of cancer*. New York: Scribner.

Musselman, D.L., Miller, A.H., Porter, M.R., Manatunga, A., Gao, F., Penna, S., . . . Nemeroff, C.B. (2001). Higher than normal plasma interleukin-6 concentrations in cancer patients with depression: preliminary findings. *American Journal of Psychiatry*, August, 158 (8): 1252–1257.

Mynors-Wallis, L. & Lau, M. (2010). Problem solving as a low intensity intervention. In *Oxford guide to low intensity CBT interventions*, 151–158 (J. Bennett-Levy et al., Eds.). Oxford, UK: Oxford University Press.

National Institute for Clinical Excellence. (2009). *Depression: management of depression in primary and secondary care*. Clinical Guideline (updated), 23. London: Department of Health.

Needleman, L. (1999). *Cognitive case conceptualization: a guidebook for practitioners*. Mahwah, NJ: Erlbaum.

Nekolaichuk, C., Watanabe, S., & Beaumont, C. (2008). The Edmonton symptom assessment system: a 15-year retrospective review of validation studies (1991–2006). *Palliative Medicine*, 22: 111–122.

Newman, C. (2013). *Core competencies in cognitive-behavioral therapy*. New York: Routledge/Taylor & Francis.

Nezu, A., Nezu, C., & D'Zurilla, T. (2007). *Solving life's problems: a 5-step guide to enhanced well-being*. New York: Springer.

Nezu, A., Nezu, C., & D'Zurilla, T. (2012). *Problem-solving therapy: a treatment manual*. New York: Springer.

Nezu, A., Nezu, C., Friedman, S., Faddis, S., & Houts, P. (1999). *Helping cancer patients cope: a problem-solving approach*. Washington, DC: American Psychological Association Press.

Nezu, A., Nezu, C., & Jain, D. (2005). *The emotional wellness way to cardiac health*. Oakland, CA: New Harbinger Press.

Nhat Hanh, T. (2001). *Old path white clouds: walking in the footsteps of the Buddha*. New York: Parallax Press.

Norcross, J. & Lambert, M. (2013). Evidence-based therapy relationships. In *Psychotherapy relationships that work: evidence-based responsiveness (2nd Edition)*, 3–21 (J. Norcross, Ed.). Oxford: Oxford University Press.

Ofri, D. (2005). *Incidental findings*. New York: Random House.

Olfson, M., Mojtabai, R., Sampson, N.A., Hwang, I., Druss, B., Wang, P.S., . . . Kessler, R.C. (2009). Dropout from outpatient mental health care in the United States. *Psychiatric Services*, 60: 898–907.

Padesky, C. (1993). *Socratic questioning: changing minds or guiding discovery?* Invited keynote address, European Congress of Behavioural and Cognitive Therapies, London.

Padesky, C. (1996). Developing cognitive therapist competency: teaching and supervision models. In *Frontiers of cognitive therapy*, 266–292 (P.M. Salkovskis, Ed.). New York: Guilford Press.

Padesky, C. & Mooney, K. (2012). Strength-based cognitive-behavioural therapy: a four-stage model for building resilience. *Clinical Psychology and Psychotherapy*, 19: 283–290.

Pasquini, M., Speca, A., Mastroeni, S., Chiaie, R., Sternberg, C., & Biondi, M. (2008). Differences in depressive thoughts between major depressive disorder, IFN-alpha-induced depression, and depressive disorders among cancer patients, *Journal of Psychosomatic Research*, August, 65 (2): 153–156.

Perri, M., Nezu, A., McKelvey, W., Shermer, R., Renjilian, D., & Viegener, B. (2001). Relapse prevention training and problem-solving therapy in the long-term management of obesity. *Journal of Consulting and Clinical Psychology*, August, 69 (4): 722–726.

Persons, J. (1989). *The case formulation approach to cognitive-behavior therapy*. New York: Guilford Press.

Persons, J. (2008). *The case formulation approach to cognitive-behavior therapy (2nd Edition)*. New York: Guilford Press.

Ramnero, J. & Toerneke, N. (2008). *The ABC's of human behavior: behavioral principles for the practicing clinician*. Oakland, CA: New Harbinger.

Ricard, M. (2015). *Altruism: the power of compassion to change yourself and the world*. New York: Little, Brown & Company.

Richards, D. (2010). Behavioral activation. In *Oxford guide to low intensity CBT interventions*, 141–150 (J. Bennett-Levy et al., Eds.), Oxford, UK: Oxford University Press.

Riskind, J., Rector, N., & Taylor, S. (2012). Looming cognitive vulnerability to anxiety and its reduction in psychotherapy. *Journal of Psychotherapy Integration*, 22 (2): 137–162.

Robichaud, M. & Dugas, M. (2006). A cognitive behavioral treatment targeting intolerance of uncertainty. In *Worry and its psychological disorders: theory, assessment and treatment*, 289–304 (G.C.L. Davey & A. Wells, Eds.). Chichester, UK: John Wiley & Sons.

Rogers, C. (1951). *Client-centered therapy: its current practice, implications, and theory*. London: Constable.

Rogers, C. (1980). *A way of being*. Boston: Houghton Mifflin.

Rolland, J. (1990). *Families, illness, & disability: an integrative treatment model*. New York: Basic Books.

Rosenberg & McDaniel. (2014). *Brief FT for med pts.*

Rost, A., Wilson, K., Buchanan, E., Hidebrandt, M., & Mutch, D. (2012). Improving psychological adjustment among late-stage ovarian cancer patients: examining the role of avoidance in treatment. *Cognitive and Behavioral Practice,* 19: 508–517.

Rouleau, C., Garland, S., & Carlson, L. (2015). The impact of mindfulness-based interventions on symptom burden, positive psychological outcomes, and biomarkers in cancer patients. *Cancer Management Research,* 7: 121–131.

Safran, J. & Segal, Z. (1990). *Interpersonal processes in cognitive therapy.* New York: Basic Books.

Salkovskis, P. (1996a). The cognitive approach to anxiety: threat beliefs, safety-seeking behavior, and the special case of health anxiety and obsessions. In *Frontiers of cognitive therapy,* 48–74 (P. Salkovsis, Ed.). New York: Guilford Press.

Salkovskis, P. (1996b). Cognitive therapy and Aaron T. Beck. In *Frontiers of cognitive therapy,* 531–539 (P. Salkovsis, Ed.). New York: Guilford Press.

Salmon, P., Clark, L., McGrath, E., & Fisher, P. (2015). Screening for psychological distress in cancer: renewing the research agenda. *Psycho-Oncology,* 24: 262–268.

Sapolsky, R. (2004). *Why zebras don't get ulcers (3rd Edition).* New York: Holt.

Schwartz, M.D., Lerman, C., Audrain, J., Cella, D., Rimer, B., Stefanek, M., . . . Vogel, V. (1998). The impact of a brief problem-solving training intervention for relatives of recently diagnosed breast cancer patients. *Annals of Behavioral Medicine,* 20 (1): 7–12.

Segal, Z., Williams, M., & Teasdale, J. (2001). *Mindfulness-based cognitive therapy for depression (1st Edition).* New York: Guilford Press.

Segal, Z., Williams, M., & Teasdale, J. (2013). *Mindfulness-based cognitive therapy for depression (2nd Edition).* New York: Guilford Press.

Seligman, M. (2011). *Flourish.* New York: Simon & Schuster.

Seligman, M. & Csikszentmilhayi, M. (2000). Positive psychology. *American Psychologist,* 55: 5–14.

Seligman, M., Steen, T., Park, N., & Peterson, C. (2005). Positive psychology progress: empirical validation of interventions. *American Psychologist,* 60: 410–421.

Shenk, C. & Fruzzetti, A. (2011). The impact of validating and invalidating responses on emotional reactivity. *Journal of Social and Clinical Psychology,* 30 (2): 163–183.

Singer, T. & Bolz, M. (2013). *Compassion: bridging science and practice.* e-book, Munich: Max Planck Institute. iBooks. https://itun.es/us/iOvrX.l

Skinner, B.F. (1957). *Verbal behavior.* Acton, MA: Copley.

Speca, M., Carlson, L., Goodey, E., & Angen, M. (2000). A randomized, wait-list controlled clinical trial: the effects of a mindfulness-based stress reduction program on mood and symptoms of stress in cancer outpatients. *Psychosomatic Medicine,* 63: 613–622.

Spivack, G., Platt, J., & Shure, M. (1976). *The problem-solving approach to adjustment.* San Francisco, CA: Jossey-Bass.

Stanton, A., Bower, J., & Low, C. (2006). Posttraumatic growth after cancer. In *Handbook of posttraumatic growth: research and practice*, 138–175 (L. Calhoun & R. Tedeschi, Eds.). New York: Psychology Press/Taylor & Francis Group.

Stanton, A., Rowland, J., & Ganz, P. (2015). Life after diagnosis and treatment of cancer in adulthood: contributions from psychosocial oncology research. *American Psychologist*, 70 (2): 159–174.

State of Mind. (2012). Interview with Tom Borkovec–EABCT 2012 Genève. [video file]. Retrieved from https://www.youtube.com/watch?v=zY9Pa1UKDrU

Stewart, B. & Wild, C. (Eds). (2014). *World cancer report*. International Agency for Research on Cancer Lyon, France: IARC Press.

Stoddard, J. & Afari, N. (2014). *The big book of ACT metaphors*. Oakland, CA: New Harbinger Press.

Stoffers, J., Völlm, B., Rucker, G., Timmer, A., Huband, N., & Lieb, K. (2012). Psychological therapies for people with borderline personality disorder. *Cochrane Library*, August 15. John Wiley & Sons. DOI: 10.1002/14651858.CD005652.pub2

Stott, R., Mansell, W., Salkovskis, P., Lavender, A., & Cartwright-Hatton, S. (2010). *Oxford guide to metaphors in CBT: building cognitive bridges*. Oxford: Oxford University Press.

Strosahl, K. & Robinson, P. (2008). *The mindfulness & acceptance workbook for depression: using acceptance & commitment therapy to move through depression and create a life worth living*. Oakland, CA: New Harbinger.

Strosahl, K., Robinson, P., & Gustavvson, T. (2012). *Brief interventions for radical change: principles and practices of focused acceptance and commitment therapy*. Oakland, CA: New Harbinger.

Strosahl, K., Robinson, P., & Gustavvson, T. (2015). *Inside this moment: a clinicians' guide to promoting radical change using acceptance and commitment therapy*. Oakland, CA: Context Press/New Harbinger.

Stuart, S. & Robertson, M. (2012). *Interpersonal psychotherapy: a clinician's guide (2nd Edition)*. Boca Raton, FL: CRC Press/Taylor Francis Group.

Talmon, M. (1990). *Single session therapy*. San Francisco, CA: Jossey-Bass.

Teasdale, J. (1993). Emotion and two kinds of meaning: cognitive therapy and applied cognitive science. *Behaviour Research and Therapy*, 31: 339–354.

Teasdale, J. (1999). Emotional processing, three modes of mind and the prevention of relapse in depression. *Behaviour Research and Therapy*, 37: 53–77.

Teasdale, J. & Chaskalson, M. (2011a). How does mindfulness transform suffering? I: the nature and origins of dukkha. *Contemporary Buddhism*, 12 (1): 89–102.

Teasdale, J. & Chaskalson, M. (2011b). How does mindfulness transform suffering? II: the transformation of dukkha. *Contemporary Buddhism*, 12 (1): 103–124.

Teasdale, J., Segal, Z., & Williams, J. (1995). How does cognitive therapy prevent depressive relapse and why should attentional control (mindfulness) training help? *Behaviour Research and Therapy*, 33 (1): 25–39.

Tedeschi, R. & Calhoun, L. (1996). The posttraumatic growth inventory: measuring the positive legacy of trauma. *Journal of Traumatic Stress*, 9 (3): 455–471.

Thompson, E. (2015). *Waking, dreaming, being: self and consciousness in neuroscience, meditation, and philosophy*. New York: Columbia University Press.

Tirch, D., Schoendorff, B., & Silberstein, L. (2014). *The ACT practitioner's guide to the science of compassion: tools for fostering psychological flexibility*. Oakland, CA: New Harbinger Press.

Toerneke, N. (2010). *Learning RFT: an introduction to relational frame theory and its clinical applications*. Oakland: New Harbinger.

Traeger, L., Greer, J., Fernandez-Robles, C., Temel, J., & Pirl, W. (2012). Evidence-based treatment of anxiety in patients with cancer. *Journal of Clinical Oncology*, 30 (11): 1197–1207.

Trask, P. (2004). Assessment of depression in cancer patients. *Journal of the National Cancer Institute Monograph*, 32: 80–92.

Van't Spijer, A., Trijsburg, R., & Duivenvoorden, H. (1997). Psychological sequelae of cancer diagnosis: a meta-analytic review of 58 studies after 1980. *Psychosomatic Medicine*, 59 (3): 280–293.

Villatte, J., Villatte, M., & Hayes, S. (2012). A naturalistic approach to transcendence: deictic framing, spirituality, and prosociality. In *The self and perspective taking: contributions and applications from modern behavioral science*, 199–216 (L. McHugh & I. Stewart, Eds.). Oakland, CA: New Harbinger Publications.

Villatte, M., Villatte, J., & Hayes, S. (2016). *Mastering the clinical conversation: language as intervention*. New York: Guilford Press.

Walsh, F. (2006). *Strengthening family resilience*. New York: Guilford Press.

Wampold, B. & Imel, Z. (2015). *The great psychotherapy debate*. New York: Routledge/Taylor & Francis.

Waraich, P., Goldner, E., Somers, J., & Hsu, L.(2004). Prevelance and incidence studies of mood disorders: a systematic review of the literature. *Canadian Journal of Psychiatry*, 49: 124–138.

Watzlawick, P. (1993). *The situation is hopeless, but not serious*. New York: W.W. Norton.

Watzlawick, P., Weakland, J., & Fisch, R. (1974). *Change: principles of problem formation and problem resolution*. New York: W.W. Norton.

Weishaar, M. (1993). *Aaron T. Beck*. London: Sage.

Wells, A. (2000). *Emotional disorders & metacognition: innovations in cognitive therapy*. London: John Wiley & Sons.

Wells, A. (2009). *Metacognitive therapy for anxiety and depression*. New York: Guilford Press.

Wells, A. & Fisher, P. (2016a). Preface. In *Treating depression: MCT, CBT and Third Wave therapies*, ix–xi (A. Wells & P. Fisher, Eds.). West Sussex, UK: John Wiley & Sons.

Wells, A. & Fisher, P. (2016b). Metacognitive therapy: theoretical background and model of depression. In *Treating depression: MCT, CBT and Third Wave therapies*, 144–168 (A. Wells & P. Fisher, Eds.). West Sussex, UK: John Wiley & Sons.

Westbrook, D., Kennerley, H., & Kirk, J. (2012). *An introduction to cognitive-behavior therapy: skills and applications.* London: Sage.

Williams, M., Fennell, M., Barnhofer, T., Crane, R., & Silverton, S. (2015). *Mindfulness and the transformation of despair: working with people at risk of suicide.* New York: Guilford Press.

Williams, N., Storey, L., & Wilson, K. (2015). Psychological interventions for patients with cancer: psychological flexibility and the potential utility of acceptance and commitment therapy, *European Journal of Cancer Care,* 24 (1): 15–27.

Wills, F. (2009). *Beck's cognitive therapy.* New York: Routledge/Taylor Francis Group.

Wills, F. (2015). *Skills in cognitive behaviour therapy (2nd Edition).* London: Sage.

Wills, F. & Sanders, D. (2013). *Cognitive behaviour therapy: foundations for practice.* London: Sage.

Wilson, K. & DuFrene, T. (2009). *An acceptance and commitment therapy approach to mindfulness in psychotherapy.* Oakland, CA: New Harbinger Press.

Wilson, K., Bordieri, M., & Whiteman, K. (2012). The self and mindfulness. In *The self and perspective taking: contributions and applications from modern behavioral science,* 181–197 (L. McHugh & I. Stewart, Eds.). Reno, NV: Context Press.

Wilson, K.G., Sandoz, E.K., Kitchens, J., & Riberts, M.(2010). The Valued Living Questionnaire: defining and measuring valued action within a behavioral framework. *The Psychological Record,* 60: 249–272.

Winnicott, D. (1987). *Child, the family and the outside world.* London: Addison Wesley.

Yalom, I. (1980). *Existential psychotherapy.* New York: Basic Books.

Young, J. & Beck, A. (1980). *Cognitive therapy scale rating manual.* Philadelphia, PA: Center for Cognitive Therapy.

Zettle, R. (2007). *ACT for depression: a clinician's guide to using acceptance & commitment therapy in treating depression.* Oakland, CA: New Harbinger.

Zettle, R. (2016). Acceptance and commitment therapy of depression. In *Treating depression: MCT, CBT and Third Wave therapies,* 169–193 (A. Wells & P. Fisher, Eds.). West Sussex, UK: John Wiley & Sons.

Index

Printed in the United States
by Baker & Taylor Publisher Services